Clinical Problem Solving for Physician Assistants

Clinical Problem Solving for Physician Assistants

Edited by

J. Dennis Blessing, PhD, PA-C

Associate Professor and Chair
Department of Physician Assistant Studies
Executive Director
Center for Allied Health Research
School of Allied Health Sciences
The University of Texas Health Science Center at San Antonio
San Antonio, Texas

 F. A. Davis Company • Philadelphia

F. A. Davis Company
1915 Arch Street
Philadelphia, PA 19103

Printed in the United States of America

Last digit indicates print number: 10 9 8 7 6 5 4 3 2 1

Acquisitions Editor: Margaret M. Biblis
Developmental Editor: Renee A. Gagliardi
Cover Designer: Louis Forgione

As new scientific information becomes available through basic and clinical research, recommended treatments and drug therapies undergo changes. The author(s) and publisher have done everything possible to make this book accurate, up to date, and in accord with accepted standards at the time of publication. The authors, editors, and publisher are not responsible for errors or omissions or for consequences from application of the book, and make no warranty, expressed or implied, in regard to the contents of the book. Any practice described in this book should be applied by the reader in accordance with professional standards of care used in regard to the unique circumstances that may apply in each situation. The reader is advised always to check product information (package inserts) for changes and new information regarding dose and contraindications before administering any drug. Caution is especially urged when using new or infrequently ordered drugs.

Library of Congress Cataloging in Publication Data

Clinical problem solving for physician assistants / edited by J. Dennis Blessing.
    p. cm.
  Includes bibliographical references and index.
  ISBN 0-8036-0769-5 (pbk.)
    1. Physician assistants. 2. Clinical competence. 3. Medical assistants. 4. Problem solving.   I. Blessing, J. Dennis.

  R728.8 .C564 2001
  610.69'53—dc21

          2001032525

*This book is dedicated
to every past, present, and future PA student
and to the teachers who guide them.
Learning is a never-ending road to the future
and each step is a life reward.*

Contributors

EDITOR

J. Dennis Blessing, PhD, PA-C
Associate Professor and Chair
Department of Physician Assistant Studies
Executive Director
Center for Allied Health Research
School of Allied Health Sciences
The University of Texas Health Science Center at San Antonio
San Antonio, Texas

> PA Duke University, 1976
> PhD Kansas State University, 1989
> *Clinical Experience:* Family Medicine, Rural Medicine, Emergency Medicine, Surgery, Transplantation, Urology, Native American General Medicine, Indigent Care

AUTHORS

Salah Ayachi, PhD, PA-C
Associate Professor
The University of Texas Medical Branch
School of Allied Health Sciences
Department of Physician Assistant Studies
Galveston, Texas

> PhD Texas A&M University, 1974
> PA The University of Texas Medical Branch, 1992
> *Clinical Experience:* HIV–Infectious Disease, Correctional Medicine

Roberto Canales, MS, PA-C
Assistant Professor
The University of Texas Medical Branch
School of Allied Health Sciences
Department of Physician Assistant Studies
Galveston, Texas

> PA The University of Texas Medical Branch, 1989
> MS The University of Texas Medical Branch, 1998
> *Clinical Experience:* Correctional Medicine, HIV–Infectious Disease,
>   Internal Medicine, In-Patient Internal Medicine

Frances Coulson, MS, PA-C
Assistant Professor
The University of Texas Medical Branch
School of Allied Health Sciences
Department of Physician Assistant Studies
Galveston, Texas

> PA The University of Texas Medical Branch, 1993
> MS The University of Texas Medical Branch, 1998
> *Clinical Experience:* Emergency Medicine, Community Health Center,
>   Correctional Medicine

Barbara A. Lyons, MA, PA-C
Associate Professor
The University of Texas Medical Branch
School of Allied Health Sciences
Department of Physician Assistant Studies
Galveston, Texas

> PA Baylor College of Medicine, 1979
> MA The University of Houston, 1986
> *Clinical Experience:* Research, Obstetrics and Gynecology

Bruce Niebuhr, PhD
Associate Professor
The University of Texas Medical Branch
School of Allied Health Sciences
Department of Physician Assistant Studies
Galveston, Texas

> PhD Southern Illinois University, 1976
> *Clinical Experience:* Experimental Psychologist

Richard R. Rahr, EdD, PA-C
Professor and Chair
The University of Texas Medical Branch
School of Allied Health Sciences
Department of Physician Assistant Studies
Galveston, Texas

> PA The University of Texas Medical Branch, 1975
> EdD The University of Houston, 1987
> *Clinical Experience:* General Internal Medicine, Geriatrics

Virginia A. Rahr, EdD, ANP
Associate Professor
School of Nursing
The University of Texas Medical Branch
Galveston, Texas

> BRN The University of Texas Medical Branch, 1970
> EdD Nova University, 1980
> ANP The University of Texas Medical Branch, 1996
> *Clinical Experience:* Adult Health, Oncology

Karen S. Stephenson, MS, PA-C
Associate Professor
The University of Texas Medical Branch
School of Allied Health Sciences
Department of Physician Assistant Studies
Galveston, Texas

> PA The University of Texas Medical Branch, 1978
> MS The University of Texas Medical Branch, 1995
> *Clinical Experience:* Rural Primary Care Medicine, Pediatrics, Indigent
> Care

Reviewers

Eleanor Babonis, PA-C
Director, Physician Assistant
    Program
King's College
Wilkes-Barre, Pennsylvania

Matt Dane Baker, PA-C, MS
Program Director
Physician Assistant Program
Philadelphia University
Philadelphia, Pennsylvania

**Richard E. Davis, MS, PA-C,
EdD(c)**
Director, Physician Assistant
    Program
Associate Dean, College of Allied
    Health
Nova Southeastern University
Fort Lauderdale, Florida

JoAnn Deasy, PA-C, MPH
Director, Physician Assistant
    Program
Catholic Medical Center
Flushing, New York

Michael Dryer, PA-C, MPH
Chair and Program Director
Physician Assistant Program
Beaver College
Glenside, Pennsylvania

Rudolph H. Duiker, AAS, BA, SPA
Academic Coordinator
Surgical Physician Assistant
    Program
Cuyahoga Community College
Parma, Ohio

Beverly Lassiter-Brown, PA-C
Chair, Physician Assistant Program
School of Medicine and Science
Charles Drew University
Los Angeles, California

Cynthia Lord, PA-C
Professor
Physician Assistant Program
Quinnipiac University
Hamden, Connecticut

Contents

Introduction to Problem-Based Learning

J. DENNIS BLESSING, PhD, PA-C

Problem-based learning (PBL) is becoming one of the dominant methods of instruction in the health professions. PBL is not new, but it is being perfected continually. PBL attempts to engage learners in a method of problem solving that will be similar to the approach they will use in practice. Being presented with problems in a practical and realistic format allows students to practice the process of diagnosis while also gaining knowledge. Learning based on problem solving provides a basis for lifelong and improved learning.

PBL has its foundations in adult learning (Table I–1) but incorporates concepts from various teaching and learning theories. The basic principles of adult learning are defined by the term androgogy (the art and science of teaching adults), or education as a tool for self-actualization, and that process should lead to the development of critical thinking.[1,2,3] At its base, androgogy contends that adults have a different set of driving forces, abilities, and experiences that should make learning a desired event that the learner partly controls.

The following are key concepts of PBL:[2]

- *Cumulative learning:* Learning is not compartmentalized. The process builds on everything that you do and learn.
- *Integrated learning:* Problems are interrelated, with mental, physical, and social implications that you must consider as a whole, *not* as separate issues or concepts.
- *Progressive learning:* As you develop as a problem solver, your skills and abilities will increase, allowing you to face more complex challenges. Evaluation of the application of learning is an important tool in student assessment.

TABLE I–1   CHARACTERISTICS OF ADULT LEARNERS[1]

- *The Learner Is Self-Directed:* Adult learners are responsible for their learning. They should be able to understand the objectives of their learning and direct themselves accordingly.
- *The Learner Is Experienced:* Adult learners come to the learning experience with broad experience and understanding of the world that they can apply to that learning experience.
- *The Learner Is Ready to Learn:* Adult learners are ready to learn. They enter the learning experience for a reason or to meet a need. Having a need or reason should be the impetus for them to learn.
- *The Learner Is Oriented to Learn:* Adult learners are oriented to learn because of a need in their life situation. They have life experiences as adults with tasks to be completed that will lead them to their goals. Those goals, tasks, or problems to be solved support their orientation to learn. They have a reason to learn.
- *The Learner Is Motivated to Learn:* Adult learners have both internal and external motivators for learning. External motivators include a desire for advancement, salary potential, a better job, and so forth. The internal motivators are stronger. These may include a desire to serve those in need or to improve one's own self-esteem or self-actualization.

- *Consistent learning:* Teachers and students can use PBL in every part of a curriculum to develop desired skills.

Your approach to PBL can assume many forms, including formal and informal learning events, individual and group efforts, multidisciplinary interactions, direction from faculty or students, high or low levels of faculty facilitation, and use of every known form of published information and data. PBL literally will take on whatever format you choose. What is important is the development of a process that will help both student and practitioner provide the best possible medical care.

PBL is learning how to learn. In writing this book, we authors had several goals for our students, which are listed in Table I–2. We hope that this book will provide a basis and stimulus for learning. We have provided direction through step-by-step case development and directed tasks. You can and should certainly go beyond these directed tasks. You must understand that this book is *not* a medical textbook or reference. Medical advances occur almost daily, so specific treatments, medications, laboratory tests, and other variables may change from those found in this book. But such changes should not affect your ability to use these cases because you will seek the most recent medical data about the problem from your library, texts, journals, the Internet, and MEDLINE. Use many resources as you work through these cases. Do not accept any one line of thought until you have explored many.

We have not covered every aspect of these cases or every approach to them. Nor have we created this book to serve as a medical reference for the cases. Doing so would be next to impossible without creating a giant tome that you probably would not want to read. The overall approach to the problem is most important, not the specific details.

TABLE I–2   GOALS FOR PROBLEM-BASED LEARNING

- To provide a basis for developing a problem-solving process
- To develop a lifelong learning framework for problem solving
- To develop an ability to find and use information
- To begin to analyze and synthesize information
- To develop an inclusive understanding of the patient and the problem
- To develop an appreciation of the costs and effects of health care
- To learn to work in a group and as an individual
- To consider medicine and health in the broadest sense and concepts
- To develop or further skills as a clinician
- To develop an ability to adapt to future changes in medicine
- To learn how to learn and to think critically about medical problems

HOW TO USE THIS BOOK

We, the authors of this text, have been involved with PBL for many years and have used case studies in particular. We have based all the cases on real patients encountered in our various practices; however, we have changed the patients' names to protect their identities.

Our recommendations for using this book are listed here, but you can use any approach you choose. Of course, if you are a student, a faculty member may direct your approach.

1. *Work in small groups,* with individuals assigned to specific components of the problem. There can be role-playing: One person can be the patient, another can act as the provider, and other group members can critique or comment. Members of the group can divide tasks. For example, one person can search the literature for the latest data on a disease, while another person can investigate costs of medications, laboratory tests, or other studies. One person can find out if Medicare or Medicaid covers a desired study or hospitalization, while another person can seek billing information and coding. One person can find information about effective alternative therapies, while another person can identify what a health maintenance organization (HMO) will cover. The tasks that your group may add to this list are unlimited. The important point is that all participate and improve their own (and the group's) problem-solving abilities. An added benefit is that you also will learn about medicine. If you use current sources of information, what you will learn will be more recent than what was available when we developed this book.

2. *Take your time,* and work through the problems completely. Go beyond just answering the questions we pose. Some cases will take multiple

sessions. You begin, go out and gather information, and meet again to add to the case solution. It is better to do a thorough job with one case than a superficial job on all of them.

3. *Consider the human factors* in each case. Put yourself in the patient's place. How would you feel? Consider the costs of what you want to do. How much does that laboratory test or diagnostic study cost? How much technology is really needed? When is magnetic resonance imaging (MRI) or computed tomography (CT) necessary? Does where the person lives, the work the person does, or the family situation influence your decision making and care? How do your decisions affect the patient and the family? Seek to enhance the patient's mental, social, and physical well-being.

4. *Review the anatomy, physiology, and pathophysiology* for all the organ systems involved with the disease process presented. You must know the anatomy and understand the physiology and pathophysiology of disease to assess and manage any problem.

5. *Seek answers from all available resources* rather than just relying on the text. Write down the answers to the questions. Add to and subtract from your answers as your knowledge increases from self-study and the input of others in your group.

6. *Develop an understanding of the warning signs of hidden and unusual problems.* All these cases are based on common problems, so they represent the types of things many of you will see in practice. Uncommon diseases do present sometimes, however, and you should learn to recognize them. Again, the medical literature coupled with your sense of inquiry is the key.

7. *Ask many questions.* Seek multiple resources to find the answers to the questions presented and to those that come up in your discussions. Discuss, consider, and debate the problems and their resolutions. Learn from individual study and from others. Challenge and stimulate one another. Challenge conventional wisdom as necessary until you are sure of what is right and accurate. Remember, we have not answered all the questions posed within each case. It is your job to answer the questions and verify those answers. Everything you do provides you with experience for your future.

It is easy to read completely through these cases and use the information given to work through them. That approach will have little value. Complete the tasks presented, and answer questions without looking ahead to the rest of the case. Use other resources in your quest for information and knowledge. Information from a single source that matches your problem exactly will not be available in your future practice, so use these cases to develop a sense of how to get the information you need and how to apply it to the problems your patients will have.

We hope that this effort will help each of you to become an excellent clinician and a lifelong learner who will serve and benefit humankind.

Note to Faculty

We have designed these cases to lead students through a process that mimics clinical interactions. Students should actively seek the information and data that will allow them to develop a sense of how to solve clinical problems. You can teach and facilitate learning, but your emphasis should be on student exploration. Do not provide the answers, but view yourself as a facilitator to the acquisition of knowledge. One method that we have found useful in problem-solving groups is to pose questions that help establish the group's directions, investigations, and energy, and then to let the group proceed on its own. Straying in many directions is acceptable; you may need to redirect students, but they will learn something from every blind or different alley. Ultimately, you will impart your knowledge to your students, but let students do as much work as possible. Do not let students rely on simple or set responses and answers. Challenge them to think.

Encourage students to explore beyond just learning signs, symptoms, and treatments. Help them to understand the effects of disease on individuals, families, and society. Encourage discussions of ethical, legal, and moral issues involved in patient care. You may want to discuss issues related to costs, third-party payers, referrals, consultation with supervising physicians, and the host of other considerations that involve today's health-care and physician assistant (PA) practice. Use these cases to benefit your students in a way that meets your program's needs and mission. Remember that these cases are templates: You can add to and expand upon them. You can make them more challenging by adding indications of other diseases or intensifying signs and symptoms. Because this is not a medical text, it does not supply every piece of information. Teach your students as they develop questions and explore problems. Use these cases in a way that helps your students to learn.

Note to the Practicing PA

Working through these cases can help you to prepare for the certifying examination or can serve as a tool for review and learning. The cases and their format may serve as a tool for self-evaluation, helping you to assess your processing of and approach to problems. The cases may validate what you already do, or they may spur you to re-evaluate your problem-solving abilities. The cases presented are common problems in primary care, but patients with similar problems will also appear in specialty practices. We believe that periodic review is valuable to every PA and hope that these cases will benefit you.

REFERENCES

1. Knowles MS, et al. *Androgogy in Action: Applying Modern Principles of Adult Learning.* San Francisco: Jossey-Bass; 1984.
2. Engel CE. In Boud D, Feletti G, eds. *The Challenge of Problem Based Learning.* New York: St. Martin's Press; 1991:29.
3. Kidd JR. *How Adults Learn.* New York: Cambridge Press; 1973:147–192.

"I Need a Checkup."

BARBARA A. LYONS, MA, PA-C

BACKGROUND

You work in a family medicine clinic.

PATIENT HISTORY

Charles Miller, a 45-year-old white man, is new to your practice. He has been married to his wife, Patricia, for 20 years. Charles and Patricia have two children: Angie, 14 years old, and Jonathan, 6 years old. The family lives in a suburb of a large city and prefers to see neighborhood health-care providers. The family is generally well, except that Angie has been "acting out" during her teenage years, which is placing great stress on her parents.

Charles's chief complaint is that he needs a physical examination (PE) because he is finishing the last steps toward admittance into the partnership of his law firm. He has not had a PE in at least 15 years. During that time, he has received treatment for any illness at an urgent care clinic in your town, but he has had no regular medical care. He says that he is generally healthy except for a few bouts of "flu" and sinusitis over the years, for which he received treatment.

T A S K S

1. What additional history do you want to know?

2. How could this patient's family life and work life contribute to any health problems he may have?

3. What social (including sexual) history do you want to obtain?

4. What are the standards for a periodic examination for a man his age?

ADDITIONAL HISTORY

The patient has been happily married for 20 years. Patricia has a part-time job at the local quilting supply store and sometimes teaches quilting classes there. Husband and wife have divided their household duties: Patricia handles the children and the house, and Charles takes care of the bills, cars, and yard. Charles works long hours (often until 8 or 9 PM) Monday through Friday and goes to the office one weekend morning each week. He has followed this routine for the past few years leading up to the partnership offer. During this time, Angie has begun to have problems. She has been caught smoking on school grounds and was suspended from school because of repeated acts of vandalism. Jonathan has been a joy to the family. A quick learner, he started reading before entering kindergarten. He is very sociable and makes friends easily. Patricia prefers to spend time with Jonathan because doing so is much more pleasant than dealing with Angie and her problems. Charles accepts that he has to work hard and long to reach his goal and thinks that Patricia should be able to shoulder her responsibilities without his help. He is a bit perturbed that she cannot do so at this time. Patricia has taken Angie to personal counseling, but Angie's behavior has continued to deteriorate. The situation embarrasses Charles, and he wonders why he is even telling you, his health-care provider, about all his family problems.

His family history includes a 70-year-old mother who has arthritis and type 2 diabetes mellitus (DM). His father, 73 years old, has hypertension and congestive heart failure (CHF). Charles has two sisters, 41 years old and 38 years old, who are well and a brother, 43 years old, who has hypertension and is obese. Patricia, 47 years old, is in good health other than an occasional migraine headache, which she controls with medication. Patricia feels stressed by so many tasks and especially Angie's behavior. She thinks that the problem is Angie's friends. Angie has no health problems other than her behavior. Jonathan is well and without any chronic medical problems.

When he was 15 years old, Charles suffered a broken tibia from a soccer injury, which healed well. He participated in several high school and college sports but now finds very little time to exercise. He misses the camaraderie of being on a sports team and finds his work lacking in this area. He eats no breakfast, bringing a large travel container of coffee with him while commuting to his job. He drinks several additional cups of coffee during the day and switches to diet soft drinks in the afternoon. He eats a "businessman's lunch," often taking clients or potential clients to nice restaurants. For dinner, he eats whatever Patricia has saved for him. He also snacks on vending machine offerings between 6 and 7 PM when he is still at work. He drinks a few double shots of whiskey when he returns home to help relieve the stress of the day. He watches television while reading the daily mail and pays bills on the weekend day he is at home. He goes to bed at 11:30 PM, has difficulty getting to sleep, then wakes up at 3 AM, and can't get back to sleep. He has to get up at 6:15 AM to prepare for the day and be out the door before 7 AM when traffic gets heavy. His daily exercise consists of the short walk from his car to the elevator in his parking garage. He doesn't have time for anything else. On Saturday or Sunday, he does yard work. He pushes the lawn mower, edges the grass, and blows the grass clippings from the sidewalk and driveway. When he finishes these activities, he is exhausted but elated from all the exercise. He lives in an environment where yard work is a year-round requirement.

T A S K S

1. Develop a list of the health problems for which this patient is at risk based on his history.

2. What are the primary areas of emphasis for the PE?

3. What laboratory tests should you consider as part of his evaluation?

4. Is Charles at risk for any psychological problems? If yes, list them. Does he have signs or symptoms of any psychological problems at this time?

5. How would you further assess his psychological problems?

6. What part does Charles's family history play in determining his future risk of disease?

7. Does where a patient lives in the United States matter when determining his or her risks for disease? If so, which diseases are more prevalent in which locations of the country?

PHYSICAL EXAMINATION

Vital signs: Pulse 86, regular; Respirations 16, unlabored; Temperature 98°F (oral); Blood pressure 148/98, right arm, sitting; Weight 210 lb (dressed); Height 5′11″ (without shoes)

Skin: Sunburned face and forearms

Head: Normocephalic; atraumatic

Eyes: Visual acuity 20/30 OU without glasses; visual fields intact to confrontation; conjunctiva pink; sclera anicteric; evidence of pterygium at the edges of the corneas bilaterally, extending 2 mm onto the corneal surface and located at 3 and 9 o'clock; pupils equal, round, reactive to light and accommodation (PERRLA); extraocular movements intact (EOMI); funduscopic examination shows sharp disc margins, slight arterioventricular (AV) narrowing, and no AV nicking

Ears: External auditory canals (EACs) intact; tympanic membranes (TMs) intact with cone of light visible bilaterally; acuity intact using ticking watch test; Weber in midline; Rinne AC>BC

Nose: Mucosa reddish-pink with a small amount of clear discharge noted; septum midline; no sinus tenderness

Mouth/throat: Mucosa pink and well-hydrated; teeth in good repair; tongue protrudes in midline; soft palate and uvula tent upon phonation; no tonsillar enlargement

Lymph nodes: No nodes palpable in the neck, axilla, or epitrochlear areas; a few shotty nodes in the inguinal area bilaterally

Thorax/lungs: Thorax symmetrical, good expansion; lungs resonant to percussion; breath sounds normal without adventitious sounds

Cardiovascular: Quiet precordium; carotid pulses 3+ and symmetrical; apical impulse palpable at third intercostal space (ICS) at midclavicular line (MCL); S1 and S2 normal without S3, S4, murmurs, or rubs

Breasts: No enlargement, lumps, or discharge noted

Abdomen: Obese and symmetrical; bowel sounds normal; liver percussed to 12 cm at the MCL, edge smooth and nontender; splenic percussion sign negative; kidneys and spleen not palpable

Genitalia: Normal circumcised penis; descended testicles; no testicular masses or hernias

Rectal: Normal sphincter tone; prostate symmetrical, not enlarged, and without nodules; stool guaiac test results are negative

Peripheral vascular: Trace edema in the feet bilaterally; pulses intact in all areas tested and 3+

Musculoskeletal: No joint deformities; full range of motion (FROM) in hands, wrists, elbows, shoulders, spine, hips, knees, and ankles

Neurologic:

   Mental status: Tense but alert and cooperative; oriented ×3

   Cranial nerves: Grossly intact

Motor: Normal muscle bulk and tone; strength 5/5 throughout; FROM and point-to-point testing intact; gait and station normal

Sensory: Romberg test results negative; sensation intact for soft touch, sharp/dull, vibration

Reflexes: 2+ for biceps, triceps, brachioradialis, knee, and ankle bilaterally; plantar reflex response is toes going downward

T A S K S

1. Should a more complete PE have been done? If yes, what components still need to be done?

2. Redefine your list of diagnoses based on what you know.

3. What effects from sun exposure can be seen on the PE, and how can these be prevented?

4. Can blood pressure be elevated from life stress or other stresses, such as pain?

5. Which diagnostic studies should be performed?

6. What are the patient's life risk factors?

LABORATORY TESTS AND DIAGNOSTIC STUDIES

1. Total serum cholesterol level is 250 mg/dL, with high-density lipoproteins (HDLs) at 43 mg/dL and triglycerides within normal limits.
2. The results of both the complete blood count (CBC) and the urinalysis (UA) are within normal limits.

T A S K S

1. What are the most likely diagnoses based on the laboratory work?

2. Should this man undergo screening for psychiatric illness? If so, what tests could be done?

3. What problems could lifestyle modifications now prevent?

4. Do you need to counsel the patient about family issues?

5. Look up the most recent mortality data for the United States. Determine any risk factors in white men of the same age as Charles. Compare the data to determine what differences there would be in risk factors if Charles were a woman instead of a man or African American or Hispanic instead of white. If Charles were 65 years of age or older, how would his risks differ? What behaviors are linked to the risks of death most common for Charles's current age group?

6. What behavior changes would you recommend to Charles to avoid death from preventable causes?

7. Does he need an electrocardiogram (EKG) or a stress test?

8. What patient education do you want to do with this patient?

9. When will you see him in follow-up?

GENERAL DISCUSSION

A person at Charles's stage in life often experiences high levels of stress. Whether it is attaining partnership in a business, gaining tenure in teaching, or reaching the level of master mechanic, the achievement of an ultimate career goal takes work. Sometimes, family time decreases while the person is busy with career expectations. This situation can be highly stressful for the person and his or her family. Often, seeing this stage as temporary and not as a lifelong habit is helpful to all. Occasionally, however, career expectations continue to escalate, even after the person has met the ultimate career goal. This issue can be tough for some families as well as have consequences for the health of all involved.

Although controversy exists about annual and other periodic examinations, it is recognized that periodic evaluations for certain aspects of health are beneficial. Recommendations on the needed frequency and components of periodic examinations change as new data become available.

T A S K

Find a reference about periodic examinations. Discuss why the items on the periodic examinations are indicated or necessary.

Resource Notes

List all the references you used for this case.

"My Baby Has a Runny Nose, Cough, and Fever."

KAREN S. STEPHENSON, MS, PA-C

BACKGROUND

You work in a family medicine clinic in a small city surrounded by rural and farming communities.

PATIENT HISTORY

The patient, Amy Perez, is an 18-month-old Hispanic girl, whose mother brings her to the clinic and gives the history. Mrs. Perez reports that Amy became ill 5 days ago while at day care, first with rhinorrhea and then with cough. The rhinorrhea is clear. The cough initially was nonproductive, but 2 days ago Amy began to cough up yellow-green sputum. Fever began the afternoon of the third day of the illness, when day-care personnel reported Amy's rectal temperature as 102.8°F. Mrs. Perez denies that Amy has had any gastrointestinal (GI) symptoms (e.g., nausea, vomiting, or diarrhea), although Amy is eating less than usual. At night, Mrs. Perez is giving Amy an over-the-counter (OTC) cough syrup with antihistamine (recommended by a television commercial) so that Amy can sleep. She isn't giving Amy this medication during the day, however, because the preparation makes Amy drowsy.

Amy lives with both parents and her 6-year-old sister in a small farming community. Her parents are well, but her sister has begun to have similar symptoms. Mrs. Perez reports that other children at Amy's day care also have had similar symptoms.

T A S K S

1. What additional questions would you ask Mrs. Perez about Amy's condition?

2. What clinical conditions should you consider based on the initial history findings that you have obtained?

3. What are common causes of rhinorrhea?

4. Does the color of the nasal drainage indicate some possible etiologies of the rhinorrhea?

5. Would the time of the year affect the diagnoses under your consideration?

6. Are some causes of rhinorrhea unique to children?

7. What is the significance, if any, of the sputum being yellow-green?

8. Does the presence of fever with the other symptoms affect your list of possible differential diagnoses?

ADDITIONAL HISTORY

During the past 18 months, Amy has had four ear infections, all during winter months. She has responded appropriately to antibiotic treatment, with resolution of middle ear effusion about 1 month after each infection. Mrs. Perez believes that Amy was given amoxicillin for each episode. Amy has also had about nine upper respiratory infections (URIs), some of which accompanied the episodes of otitis media (OM). During Amy's current illness, Mrs. Perez has not noticed any tearing, nasal rubbing, or sneezing.

The parents use no tobacco products. There is no family history of asthma, allergies, or eczema. The family lives in a small, three-bedroom house with carpeting and no pets. Each child has her own room. Amy still sleeps in her crib, usually with dolls and stuffed animals.

Other than the URIs and OM, Amy has not been ill. Her mother denies allergies, asthma, atopic dermatitis, pneumonia, surgeries, or injuries. She states that Amy's immunizations are current. Results of her purified protein derivative (PPD) were negative at age 12 months. Amy was weaned from the bottle at 12 months and began bovine milk without problems. Her hemoglobin was 12.3 at 12 months. Her development has been normal. She speaks in two-word phrases, follows simple directions, and has a 20-word vocabulary.

Amy was the sole product of a normal pregnancy and vaginal delivery. She weighed 8 lb, 4 oz at birth and was breast-fed for the first 6 months of life. There were no major neonatal problems, although she was jaundiced secondary to breast-feeding.

T A S K S

1. What portions of the physical examination (PE) are mandatory for this child?

2. What modifications in the PE do you make for young children?

3. What are the normal values for vital signs in children this age?

4. What should this child be able to do according to the Denver Developmental II Scale?

5. What immunizations should Amy have had or does she need now?

6. Has she had an abnormal number of URIs and episodes of OM?

7. What are the risk factors for developing URIs, OM, allergy symptoms, or asthma?

8. Make a preliminary list of differential diagnoses based on the history.

PHYSICAL EXAMINATION

General: Patient sits with her mother and appears ill.

Vital signs: Pulse 130; Respirations 36; Temperature 101°F (axillary); Blood pressure not taken (she is younger than 3 years); no grunting, retractions, or nasal flaring

Skin: Warm and dry to the touch

Head: Normocephalic

Eyes: Pupils equal, round, reactive to light and accommodation (PERRLA); sclera anicteric; conjunctiva clear

Ears: External ear canals patent with some cerumen; tympanic membranes (TMs) visible, red with loss of landmarks, bulging and immobile to insufflation

Nose: Patent nares; moist and reddish mucosa; clear mucus in each nostril

Mouth: Teeth present and without cavities; mucous membranes moist

Throat: No lesions; tonsillar size enlarged 2+ with erythema but no exudate; red posterior pharynx and palate

Chest:

Inspection: No lesions; respiratory effort normal, but tachypneic; no use of accessory muscles with respiration

Auscultation: Vesicular breath sounds with some rhonchi over bronchial areas that clear with coughing; no rales or wheezing heard in any lung field

Heart: Tachycardic with regular rhythm; no murmurs, rubs, or gallops

Abdomen: Soft, protuberant, with active bowel sounds; no hepato-splenomegaly or masses felt; no rebound

Neurologic: No obvious or gross central or peripheral deficits

Extremities: Moves all extremities equally well; no cyanosis or edema noted

T A S K S

1. Refine your list of preliminary differential diagnoses based on the patient's history and PE.

2. What laboratory tests and diagnostic studies would you order?

3. Make a list of what each item in task 2 will tell you and how it will add to your assessment and management of Amy.

LABORATORY TESTS AND DIAGNOSTIC STUDIES

1. A rapid screen for streptococcus (strep screen) is done, and findings are reported as negative.
2. A tympanogram is done (Fig. 2–1).

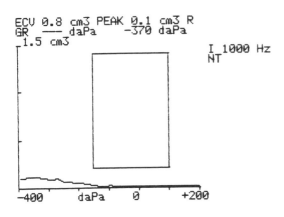

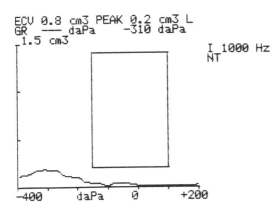

FIGURE 2–1 The tympanogram results from the evaluation of Amy Perez's TMs. The box in the center of the graph defines the normal movement of the TM. The horizontal axis measures pressures in the EAC in daPas (decapascals) from negative (−400) to positive (+200) values. The vertical axis measures compliance or movement of the TMs (changes in the volume of the EAC) in cm³. The EAC volume is represented by ECV; the normal range for a child is 0.5 to 1.2 cm³. The gradient (GR) measures the shape or width of the tracing in which the pressures and compliance are graphed against one another.

When a tympanogram is normal, the tracing will appear inside the box and will have a normal compliance (>0.2 cm³) and a normal gradient (<150 daPas). This is colloquially referred to as the "Christmas tree shape." When the gradient is >150 daPas and the compliance is <0.2 cm³, fluid fills the middle ear space (the so-called flat tympanogram). Sometimes the pressure or compliance may not be measurable because the TM is very tense from fluid accumulation in the middle ear space. When the compliance is >0.2 cm³ but the gradient is >150 daPas, the middle ear space is filled with both fluid and air. For further information about interpreting tympanograms, visit http://atc.utmb.edu/aom/tympanometry/default.htm.[10]

T A S K S

1. Use the findings of the history, PE, and laboratory and diagnostic studies to refine your final list of diagnoses.

2. What clinical clues and laboratory findings best support bacterial infection of the upper respiratory system? What findings best support viral infection? Why is it important to recognize these differences?

3. Should a throat culture be done?

4. What does the tympanogram demonstrate? Is the tympanogram normal or abnormal? What do normal and abnormal tympanograms look like?

5. How long does it take to get the results of a throat culture?

6. What do the following tests cost at your institution: rapid strep screen, throat culture, tympanogram?

DIFFERENTIAL DIAGNOSES FOR RUNNY NOSE, COUGH, AND FEVER

Consider allergies, infections, structural lesions, systemic illness (cystic fibrosis, diabetes), vasomotor or idiopathic rhinitis (exposure to irritants or change in temperature, and food allergies).[1] Common etiologies for these symptoms are:

- *Rhinitis* or *rhinopharyngitis:* Viral causes include respiratory syncytial virus (RSV), rhinovirus, influenza virus, adenovirus, parainfluenza, and enterovirus.[2]
- *Viral vesicular* or *ulcerative pharyngitis:* Herpangina (coxsackie virus), enterovirus, or herpes simplex virus.[3]
- *Pharyngoconjunctival fever:* Fever, pharyngitis, conjunctivitis, cervical adenopathy, and rhinitis; caused by adenovirus.
- *Tonsillaropharyngitis, bacterial:* Group A β-hemolytic streptococcus, pneumococcus, diphtheria, gonococcus, *Mycoplasma pneumoniae, Haemophilus influenzae.*[4]
- *Tonsillaropharyngitis, viral:* Adenovirus, Epstein-Barr virus.
- *Sinusitis, OM, or both:* Caused by various bacteria, the three most common being *Streptococcus pneumoniae, H. influenzae,* and *Moraxella catarrhalis*[5]; infrequent causes include group A streptococcus, *Staphylococcus aureus,* and gram-negative enteric bacilli.

T A S K S

1. How did you eliminate some differential diagnoses based on the information that you collected?

2. What clinical clues would lead you to consider a viral rather than a bacterial cause?

3. How will you treat this child? (Remember medication, palliative treatment, patient education, follow-up, and the need to return.)

GENERAL DISCUSSION

After consideration of the history, PE, laboratory tests, and diagnostic studies, the most likely diagnosis for this child is viral URI with bilateral OM. Fever implies that the present condition is acute rather than chronic. The nasal mucosa is reddish, not violet or pale as would be expected with allergic rhinitis. The patient's mother also has not noticed nasal itching or rubbing, and there is no family history of IgE-mediated disease. The parents have not noticed long-term (more than 7 to 10 days) rhinorrhea or any trigger factors, such as changes in the weather or exposure to pollens, pollutants, or animals. Amy still sleeps in her crib, so she does not have a large amount of bedding, although she does have carpet and stuffed animals in her room.

No ulcers, vesicles, or tonsillar exudate are noted in this child, which helps to rule out herpangina, bacterial or viral tonsillitis, and pharyngitis. If you were uncertain or exudate was present, you would perform a rapid strep screen, a culture, or both. Streptococcal pharyngitis is the most likely diagnosis when the child is aged 5 to 8 years and the predominant symptom is sore throat with dysphagia and headache, enlarged cervical lymph nodes, and fever.[6] Only about one-third of patients with streptococcal pharyngitis have enlarged tonsils with exudate and erythema.[3] Cough, rhinorrhea, hoarseness, anterior stomatitis, discrete ulcerative lesions, viral exanthems, conjunctivitis, and diarrhea point toward a viral infection.[3,6] Erythema of the throat as the only symptom usually occurs with rhinovirus, parainfluenza, RSV, influenza, or rotavirus.[3] Adenovirus and some enteroviruses usually cause cobblestone mucosa or follicular pharyngitis.[3] Enterovirus or herpes simplex virus commonly causes ulcerative or vesicular lesions.[3]

The classic pattern for OM is the onset of URI symptoms followed about 3 days later by fever, ear pain, or otorrhea. Children younger than 2 years who attend day care and have recurrent URIs are at greatest risk of developing OM.[7] The following viruses have been identified as causative for OM: RSV, parainfluenza virus, influenza virus, enteroviruses, adenoviruses, and rhinovirus.[2] It is now known that viral URIs impair host defenses in the middle ear, which enables bacteria from the nasopharynx to invade the sterile middle ear space. Examination of the ears reveals that the TMs are bulging, immobile, and cloudy. These three findings are most predictive of OM (99%), whereas a bulging, immobile, erythematous TM is 94% predictive of OM.[8] Redness is predictive of OM only when combined with bulging or immobility of the TM.

The tympanogram measures the movement of the eardrum when stimulated by sound and subjected to changes in air pressure within the external and middle ear that are produced by the tympanogram equipment. Under normal conditions, the TM will move in both directions when stimulated. If there is effusion in the middle ear, the TM will not move freely when subjected to negative or positive pressures. If both fluid and air are present in the middle ear, the TM moves more easily in a negative direction because of the negative pressure that accumulates when the eustachian tube opening in the pharynx is edematous. Because of the increased negative pressure, the TM cannot easily move in the positive direction. This pattern is expected for serous otitis (also called otitis media with effusion). The tympanogram cannot determine whether the effusion is an acute condition or whether the fluid is infected.

Amy's tympanogram (see Fig. 2–1) shows no gradient pressure and very small compliance, demonstrating that her TMs are immobile, and show that her external auditory canals (EACs) are normal in size, a pattern most consistent with OM. The tympanogram results and visualization of the TM must be used concurrently to determine whether the effusion is acutely infected or not. When fluid in the middle ear is acutely infected, the TM will generally be bulging and red. When the fluid has been there for some time, the TMs will appear gray but not bulging or red. In either of these cases, the gradient would be >150 daPas and the compliance <0.2 cm³.

The OM in this patient has had no noticeable effects on her language acquisition, as noted by her developmentally appropriate language skills. The rhinorrhea, though producing purulent material, has not been present long enough (more than 10 days) to be consistent with bacterial sinusitis.[9] The predominant aspects of this child's illness are consistent with URI: rhinorrhea, cough, and fever. Because the child's present condition includes both viral and bacterial illness, treatment should be tailored for each. There remains no indication for the administration of antibiotics to a patient with a viral illness. In this case, however, the child has a bacterial infection secondary to the viral illness. Because antibiotics were and still are being dispensed for viral illnesses, bacteria responsible for some URIs have developed resistance to many antibiotics suitable for OM or sinusitis.[7] Treatment of children in day care is complicated because of the opportunities for children to be exposed to resistant bacterial strains.

Choice of antibiotics must include those that will kill any of the three common strains, including drug-resistant and beta-lactamase–producing strains. Amoxicillin still can be given, but for children younger than 2 years, those in day care, or those who have received antibiotics in the last 3 months, the recommended dose has been increased from 40–45 mg/kg per day every 8 hours to 80–90 mg/kg per day every 8 hours.[7] In addition, a change in antibiotics must be made if there is no improvement in 48 hours. For most children, the effusion will resolve in 2 to 4 weeks without any long-term effects on hearing or language development. If the fluid persists for longer than 12 weeks or 90 days, the provider should refer the child to an ear, nose, and throat specialist for possible placement of ventilation tubes.

Palliative treatment may include antipyretics, such as acetaminophen or ibuprofen, as well as various antihistamines and decongestants. Opinions vary among health-care professionals as to the degree of benefit of such medications in easing the discomfort of upper respiratory symptoms. Very young infants should not be given decongestants and antihistamines, but a bulb syringe can be used to evacuate the nose, or saline drops can be administered to promote drainage and clearing of mucus. A review of clinical trials evaluating the use of palliative medications for URIs reveals that antipyretics are the only effective treatments.[3] Decongestants and antihistamines may cause lethargy, agitation, or cardiovascular effects. Antihistamines work for allergic rhinitis but not for URIs. Cough suppressants and decongestants may have only minimal effects, but many parents will still inquire about or choose to medicate their children with various OTC medications. None should be given to children younger than 6 months, and providers should educate parents about the effects of these OTC medications, even for older children. URIs are very common among children, and providers should take care when choosing medications for each child's condition.

REFERENCES

1. International Rhinitis Management Working Group. International Consensus Report on the diagnosis and management of rhinitis. *Allergy.* 1994;49(19 Suppl.):1–34.
2. Bluestone CD, Klein JO. *Otitis Media in Infants and Children.* 2nd ed. Philadelphia: WB. Saunders; 1995:64.
3. Herendeen NE, Szilagy PG. Infections of the upper respiratory tract. In Behrman RE, Kliegman RM, Jenson HB, eds. *Nelson Textbook of Pediatrics.* 16th ed. Philadelphia: WB Saunders; 2000:1261–1266.
4. Green M. *Pediatric Diagnosis: Interpretation of Symptoms and Signs in Children and Adolescents.* 6th ed. Philadelphia: WB Saunders; 1998:378–388.
5. Bluestone CD, Klein JO. *Otitis Media in Infants and Children.* 2nd ed. Philadelphia: WB Saunders; 1995:55.
6. Dajana A, Taubert K, Ferrieri P, et al. Treatment of acute streptococcal pharyngitis and prevention of rheumatic fever: A statement for health care professionals. *Pediatrics.* 1995;96:758–764.
7. Dowell SF, Butler JC, Giebink GS, et al. Acute otitis media: management and surveillance in an era of pneumococcal resistance—a report from the drug-resistant *Streptococcus pneumoniae* Therapeutic Working Group. *Pediatr Infect Dis J.* 1999;18:1–9.
8. Pelton SI. Otoscopy for the diagnosis of otitis media. *Pediatr Infect Dis J.* 1998;17:540–543.
9. Hueston WJ, Eberlein C, Johnson D, Mainous AG. Criteria used by clinicians to differentiate sinusitis from viral upper respiratory tract infection. *J Fam Pract.* 1998;46:487–492.
10. The University of Texas Medical Branch. Acute otitis media Web site. Patient evaluation: tympanogram. Date not available. Available at: http://atc.utmb.edu/aom/tympanometry/default.htm.

Resource Notes

List all the references you used for this case.

"My Knee Is Giving Me Fits!"

FRANCES COULSON, MS, PA-C

BACKGROUND

You work in a general medical clinic in a medium-sized city.

PATIENT HISTORY

Helen Callahan is a 67-year-old white woman and a widow. She complains of increasing soreness in her left knee for the past 2 months with occasional "near buckling." She states that she has had knee pain, right hip pain, and stiffness in both hands in the past, but her knee has been the worst problem. While she was at work recently, she slipped slightly on a wet floor but did not fall down. She has tried wearing a knee brace and taking acetaminophen, which have helped ease the pain somewhat. She has become more worried about her joint disease because her mother was almost an invalid with joint pain before she died.

T A S K S

1. What can cause joint pain?

2. What causes of joint pain have a familial or hereditary pattern?

3. What additional history should you seek, and what does each question help you determine?

4. What risk factors for joint disease are important relative to the patient's age, race, and family history?

5. Describe the anatomy of the knee joint.

ADDITIONAL HISTORY

Mrs. Callahan typically has stiffness in her knees, lower back, and hands for about 10 to 15 minutes every morning upon awakening; it improves once she gets up and about. Her knees tend to "creak" with bending, but she denies any swelling, redness, or warmth in them. The pain improves with rest, but if she sits too long, her knees stiffen. Heavy activity, such as prolonged walking and housecleaning, worsen the pain.

She has recently started working at a local store as a greeter and stands on cement for about 12 hours (4 hours × 3 days) each week. She denies actual buckling but has almost fallen on several occasions when she felt as if her knee was giving way. She denies locking in her knees and any fever, chills, or recent infections. She describes the pain as a deep ache in the joint, without radiation, and rates it 5 on a scale of 1 to 10. The pain has started interfering with her daily walk at the local mall. She denies other health problems. She takes one aspirin each day for her "circulation," as suggested by her sister. Her immunizations are current. She experienced menopause around age 56 and has had no vaginal bleeding since. She is not taking hormone replacement therapy (HRT). She has had no accidents except for falling from a horse onto her left knee when she was 17 years old. She was told it was "bruised." She had cholecystectomy at age 42 with no sequelae.

Her mother died at age 88 from a cerebrovascular accident (CVA). The mother had hypertension, "arthritis," and a bone problem that caused her to walk "hunched over" in her later years. The patient's father died at age 72 from a myocardial infarction (MI). He had other, unknown medical problems. The patient's sister is 72 years old and has hypertension and "arthritis." One brother, who had a history of alcoholism, died at age 43 in a motor vehicle collision (MVC). Three years ago, the patient's husband died at age 68 of lung cancer. Her two sons are married, and each has two children. All are healthy. One son lives in Nome, Alaska, and the other in Pittsburgh, Pennsylvania. She sees each son once or twice each year.

Mrs. Callahan finished high school, then married her high school sweetheart and worked in the home. Her husband worked for a large refinery in your city. Since her husband's death, the patient has lived alone in a house in a small nearby town. She enjoys gardening and her dog, Wag. She attends a local church regularly and has some friends she sees occasionally. She drives her car to work but does not drive at night because her vision is decreased in the dark. She eats cereal for breakfast, a salad or sandwich for lunch, and some sort of meat and vegetable for dinner. She frequently snacks at work and drinks several soft drinks each day. She had a male friend last year, but he started seeing someone else. She currently is not interested in any new relationships. She smoked two packs of cigarettes a day for 30 years but stopped about 7 years ago. She drinks one glass of wine 2 to 3 days each week with dinner. She has never used illicit drugs. She has Medicare but no supplemental insurance.

T A S K S

1. Develop a list of differential diagnoses based on the history.

2. How does the patient's medication or lack of needed medication (if any) affect her complaint?

3. How does her lifestyle affect her complaint?

4. How does her complaint affect her lifestyle?

5. How does her family history affect her complaint?

6. What effect does no HRT have? Does the patient need supplemental calcium?

7. Given that the entire physical examination (PE) is important, describe the components of the PE that are pertinent. What would you look for in each component?

PHYSICAL EXAMINATION

General: Obese woman, appropriately dressed for the season, is in no acute distress. She is alert and oriented × 3.

Vital signs: Pulse 88, regular; Respirations 18, nonlabored; Temperature 98.8°F (oral); Blood pressure 168/92, arm, sitting; Weight 188 lb; Height 5'6"

Head: Normocephalic; appropriate distribution of hair

Eyes: Pupils equal, round, reactive to light and accommodation (PERRLA); extraocular movements intact (EOMI); corneas without opacities; sclera anicteric; conjunctiva clear; mild arteriovenous (AV) nicking without hemorrhages or exudates on funduscopic examination

Ears: External auditory canals (EACs) partially occluded by cerumen with right tympanic membrane (TM) not visible; left TM pearly gray with visible landmarks and cone of light

Nose: Nares patent; mucosa pink and moist without discharge

Mouth/throat: Fair dentition with two partial plates in place; no lesions, ulcerations, or masses; tonsils not visible; posterior pharynx nonerythematous

Neck: Supple; no masses; thyroid nonpalpable

Chest: Symmetrical with normal spinal curvature; nontender to palpation; symmetrical expansion; resonant to percussion, clear to auscultation without adventitious sounds bilaterally; tactile fremitus normal; breasts equal in size and shape; skin without lesions; no masses or nipple discharge

Heart: Quiet precordium; point of maximal impulse (PMI) at fifth intercostal space (ICS) of midclavicular line (MCL); regular rate and rhythm with normal S1 and S2; no murmurs, gallops, or rubs

Abdomen: Obese; normoactive bowel sounds throughout without bruits; nontender to light and deep palpation; well-healed 12-cm scar in right upper quadrant; no masses or hepatosplenomegaly

Genitourinary: Not done

Extremities: No clubbing, cyanosis, edema, or scars; varicose veins apparent in both lower extremities; knees with full range of motion (FROM), crepitus on movement; nontender to palpation; no joint laxity, swelling, or effusion; strength 5+ bilaterally; pulses 4+ bilaterally

Neurologic: Cranial nerves I–XII grossly intact; deep tendon reflexes (DTRs) 2/4 throughout; cerebellar functions intact

T A S K S

1. List the pertinent findings (positive and negative) of the PE.

2. Redevelop your list of differential diagnoses.

3. What laboratory and diagnostic tests, procedures, and studies are appropriate for this patient? For each item, list the approximate cost and what information you expect to glean from it.

4. Are there any special PE maneuvers that you would have done (or that are indicated in the evaluation of the knee) that could add to your evaluation of her knee?

5. Should you do a pelvic and rectal examination?

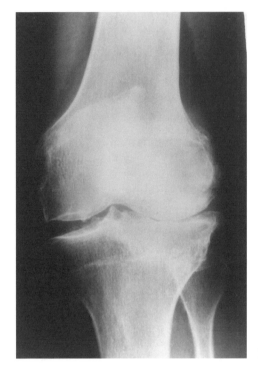

FIGURE 3–1   X-ray of knee.

LABORATORY TESTS AND DIAGNOSTIC STUDIES

1. Complete blood count (CBC) results are normal.
2. Erythrocyte sedimentation rate (ESR) is normal.
3. Blood chemistry study results are normal.
4. Urinalysis (UA) results are normal.
5. Rheumatoid factor (RF) results are negative.
6. X-ray findings are shown in Figure 3–1.

T A S K S

1. Redefine your diagnoses based on the previous information.

2. What do the x-ray results reveal?

3. Develop a treatment/management plan for each of the following causes of knee pain:
   A. Osteoarthritis/degenerative joint disease
   B. Meniscal tear
   C. Anterior cruciate ligament tear

D. Bursitis
E. Joint infection

4. What are the indications for referral to a rheumatologist or orthopedist?

5. Will physical or occupational therapy help?

6. When is joint replacement indicated?

7. Discuss and develop a treatment/management plan for the patient's other problems.

Resource Notes

List all the references you used for this case.

"I've Got the Runs!"

J. DENNIS BLESSING, PhD, PA-C

BACKGROUND

You are working in an acute care ambulatory clinic in a medium-sized city.

PATIENT HISTORY

The patient, John Nguyen, is a 36-year-old Asian man. He is a midlevel manager for a local communications company and travels quite often for his company. He is taking no regular medications, is 20 lb overweight, and is trying to diet. Previous providers have told him to watch his diet and restrict his salt intake because his blood pressure readings last year were at borderline levels for hypertension. He has no allergies.

His presenting complaint is a 2-day history of diarrhea without abdominal pain or vomiting. He has had some nausea, particularly when he has tried to eat heavy foods. He thinks he may have had a fever yesterday because he felt warm, but he did not take his temperature.

T A S K S

1. What additional history do you want to obtain? Make a list of questions.

2. What is the definition of diarrhea?

3. What is the difference between acute and chronic diarrhea?

4. What are the most common causes of acute diarrhea?

5. What are the most common causes of chronic diarrhea?

6. What are the risk factors for "traveler's diarrhea"?

7. Are any risk factors for gastrointestinal (GI) disease more common in people of Asian descent?

ADDITIONAL HISTORY

The patient had no problems or complaints until the abrupt onset of watery diarrhea with some formed elements. This began midmorning 2 days ago, and he had about eight episodes by midnight. He slept but had to get up twice in the night to go to the bathroom. He was able to eat and to drink fluids the next morning. Associated symptoms included mild nausea and subjective fever. During some episodes, he had mild abdominal cramping. He noticed no blood in the diarrhea. The next day he took two tablets of loperamide, 2 mg. Two hours later, he had an episode of diarrhea and took another 2-mg tablet of loperamide. He then had no diarrhea for 6 or 7 hours, during which he ate lunch and supper. The diarrhea returned last evening, and he has had four episodes since then. He had juice and toast for breakfast this morning.

The patient has had no previous problems with diarrhea or any other GI illness. He has not traveled outside the country. His last trip was to Las Vegas 2 weeks ago. He ate normally and had no problems while there. He had strep throat 2 months ago and took potassium penicillin for 10 days as treatment. He has eaten no raw seafood. He has not drunk water from a well. No one else at his work is ill.

Mr. Nguyen is heterosexual and has been in a monogamous relationship for the past 15 months. His partner is not ill. He has no family history of GI problems.

T A S K S

1. What is loperamide, and how does it work? What is the common dosage and treatment regimen?

2. What is the most common cause of diarrhea in all age groups?

3. Could this patient's diarrhea be antibiotic induced?

4. What symptoms would lead you to consider a chronic illness versus an acute one?

5. What are the health dangers of continued diarrhea?

6. What are the pertinent components of the physical examination (PE)?

PHYSICAL EXAMINATION

General: Patient is a well-developed, well-nourished man in no apparent distress; he answers appropriately and is oriented × 3.

Vital signs: Pulse 88; Respirations 12, regular; Temperature 99.2F° (oral); Blood pressure 138/86

Lungs: Clear to auscultation and percussion

Heart: Regular rhythm and rate; normal S1 and S2 without murmur, rubs, or gallops

Abdomen: Hyperactive bowel sounds throughout; tympanic percussion noted; mild lower quadrant tenderness without rebound; no masses; no organomegaly

Rectal examination: Not done at patient's request

T A S K S

1. Based on the information you have, develop a list of differential diagnoses.

2. Discuss whether a rectal examination should have been done.

3. What laboratory tests or other studies would you consider?

4. If you believe that the patient has viral gastroenteritis, what is the treatment? Be sure to include medications, diet, and follow-up.

5. Review each of the following common diseases that can cause diarrhea, and decide if this patient's symptoms could indicate that disease:
   A. Irritable bowel syndrome
   B. Medication-induced diarrhea

C. Lactose intolerance
D. Diverticulosis
E. Infectious diarrhea
F. Inflammatory bowel disease

RESOLUTION

A diagnosis of acute viral gastroenteritis was made. Treatment consisted of clear liquids for 24 hours, a BRAT diet for 24 hours, then a gradual increase in diet. Follow-up was scheduled for 3 to 4 days later if the diarrhea continued or worsened, or if the patient began to vomit, developed a fever above 101°F, or developed any new symptoms.

T A S K S

1. Is this the best treatment for an adult without any signs of dehydration or complicating factors?

2. Can he take over-the-counter (OTC) medications, such as loperamide, bismuth subsalicylate, or an absorbent such as kaolin and pectin?

3. Should the provider give a prescription for diphenoxylate plus atropine?

4. What does "clear liquids" mean?

5. What is the usual course of viral gastroenteritis?

6. What are the signs and symptoms that would lead to a consideration of diarrhea as a result of "food poisoning"?

7. What would your considerations and recommendations be if this patient were a child or an infant?
   A. Familiarize yourself with the recommendations for fluid replacement in children and infants.
   B. What tests are done on stool for evaluation of diarrheal disease?

8. When would you consider doing stool cultures or fecal smears or tests for ova and parasites?

9. What is a BRAT diet?

GENERAL DISCUSSION

The challenge in any patient with diarrhea, nausea, or vomiting is deciding if the etiology is viral and usually self-limiting or if you should carry out more in-depth investigations. You must be particularly careful with infants, young children, older adults, and immunocompromised patients. Hydration is very important. History questions should focus on travel, exposure to food toxins, and antibiotic use. Illnesses without the "red flags" of severity are usually managed conservatively with the primary focus on hydration.

Resource Notes

List all the references you used for this case.

"I Have a Discharge."

J. DENNIS BLESSING, PhD, PA-C • BARBARA A. LYONS, MA, PA-C

BACKGROUND

You work in a family practice clinic in a small town.

PATIENT HISTORY

Connie Janlee, a 30-year-old white woman, is the single mother of two children: a 5-year-old girl and a 10-year-old boy. Ms. Janlee's chief complaint is a vaginal discharge that began about 1 week ago. Her last menstrual period was 3 weeks ago and of normal duration and flow. Her previous menstrual period was 1 month before and normal. She has had no chronic illnesses and takes no medications. You have seen her on two or three previous occasions for mild, limited problems.

T A S K S

1. What additional history do you want?

2. List the most common causes of vaginal discharge and their characteristics.

3. What social (including sexual) history do you want?

ADDITIONAL HISTORY

Ms. Janlee has been divorced for 3 years following a 9-year marriage. During her marriage, she had sex with only her husband; however, she suspects that he cheated on her during the last year they were married. She had no other sexual partners until 2 months ago, when she started a sexual relationship with a 32-year-old man she met at church. They dated for 3 months before beginning sexual relations. She has no history of any sexually transmitted diseases (STDs) and as far as she knows, neither does her current partner. They use condoms (every time) and spermicidal jelly for birth control. They have had vaginal and oral sex.

Her discharge is thick and mostly clear to gray; it has an odor and sometimes seems worse after intercourse. She has had some mild vulvar itching. She denies other symptoms, and the review of systems (ROS) is noncontributory. She has had annual Papanicolaou tests with no abnormalities noted. The last was 9 months ago.

T A S K S

1. Based on the history you have, develop a list of differential diagnoses for this patient.

2. What are the primary areas of emphasis for your physical examination (PE)?

3. What laboratory tests should you consider as part of this patient's evaluation?

PHYSICAL EXAMINATION

Vital signs: Pulse 74; Respirations 12; Temperature 99.0°F (oral); Blood pressure 112/66; Weight 105 lb; Height 5'2"

Abdomen: Flat, active bowel sounds in all four quadrants; nontender to light and deep palpation; no masses or organomegaly

Pelvic: Vaginal mucosa pink and moist; grayish-white discharge, vulva is nonerythemic; os parous; cervix nontender to manipulation; uterus anteflexed and of normal size and consistency; adnexa nontender and without mass; ovaries normal sized and nontender bilaterally

Rectal: Confirmatory; stool occult blood negative

T A S K S

1. Should a more complete PE have been done?

2. What tests do you want to do on the discharge?

3. What other tests should you do (with the patient's permission)?

4. Redefine your list of diagnoses based on what you know.

LABORATORY TESTS AND DIAGNOSTIC STUDIES

1. Vaginal pH is 5.
2. Wet mount shows no *Trichomonas vaginalis* but numerous clue cells. KOH test produces a fishy odor, but no budding yeast or hyphae are seen.
3. DNA probe of the cervix for gonorrhea (GC) and chlamydia is done and sent to a laboratory.
4. Pregnancy test results are negative.

T A S K S

1. What is the most likely diagnosis based on the laboratory work above? Should a DNA probe for GC and chlamydia have been taken from her throat?

2. What are test "sensitivity" and "specificity"? How are they calculated, and what do they mean to you in your choice and interpretation of the tests you choose and use?

3. Should this woman be screened for human immunodeficiency virus (HIV), syphilis, hepatitis, or other STDs?

4. How often and for how long should screening for HIV and syphilis be done?

5. Do you need to counsel her on STDs or birth control?

6. Which of the following causes of vaginal discharge are considered STDs and require that the partner(s) be treated?
   A. Trichomoniasis

B. *Candida* vaginitis
C. Bacterial vaginosis
D. GC
E. Herpetic vaginitis

7. What is the treatment for each of the above?

8. Which of the above must you report to the health department or other local or state agency?

9. What forms of birth control can a 30-year-old woman use?

10. What are the risks and benefits of each type of birth control you listed?

11. What patient education do you want to do with this woman?

12. When will you see her in follow-up?

GENERAL DISCUSSION

Bacterial vaginosis (*Gardnerella vaginalis*) is the most common cause of abnormal vaginal discharge (40% to 50% of cases). Two other common causes are vulvovaginal candidiasis and trichomoniasis. Each has characteristics that point to the etiology, but evaluation without the aid of wet mounts and KOH preparations can be difficult.

Greater issues are important in this case—the risk of other STDs, particularly HIV, hepatitis, and syphilis. Even though the patient met her partner at church and they may be monogamous, the risk of STD transmission still exists. Both should be screened for HIV, hepatitis, and syphilis and counseled on future screenings. Until screening results are negative for 9 months (except for hepatitis) and neither has other sexual partners, they should use condoms. This issue can be difficult for some couples because of beliefs that STDs cannot happen to them, that condoms represent a barrier to their intimacy, that condoms interfere with sensation, and so forth.

T A S K S

1. Make a list of all the STDs you can think of, and then look up how many there are.

2. Think about and discuss in a group how you will approach sensitive issues such as STDs, birth control, and HIV/syphilis infection with your patients.

3. Practice counseling techniques and how to approach patients about sensitive issues, especially about the need for barrier protection for up to 9 months.

4. Research the recommendations of the Centers for Disease Control and Prevention (CDC) for the evaluation and treatment of STDs.

5. Discuss issues involved in patient confidentiality. This is a small town, and "the word gets around about such things."

Resource Notes

List all the references you used for this case.

"My Doc Can't Control It."

ROBERTO CANALES, MS, PA-C

BACKGROUND

You work in a family practice clinic in a large city.

PATIENT HISTORY

The patient, John Steven Collier, is a 70-year-old African-American man who comes to the clinic for an initial visit. He has recently moved from another city and brings copies of his medical records with him. He states that he has high blood pressure, adding, "My doc can't control it."

T A S K S

1. What effect does the patient's age have on his blood pressure?

2. Is the patient's age a major risk factor for hypertension?

3. Is the patient's sex a major risk factor for hypertension?

4. Does the patient's race influence his risk for complications associated with hypertension?

5. What are the risks of untreated hypertension?

6. What are the definitions for the stages of hypertension?

7. What should be done to evaluate and monitor patients with hypertension?

8. What lifestyle modifications should persons with hypertension make?

9. What categories of medications are used? When do you decide to use or to change them?

10. What additional history do you want from Mr. Collier?

ADDITIONAL HISTORY

Mr. Collier was diagnosed with essential hypertension 20 years ago and has used multiple antihypertensive medications as treatment. He is familiar with only his current medications, which he admits to skipping occasionally. He always resumes taking the pills, however, because without them "I get headaches and just feel bad." One of his main concerns is his inability to achieve full penile erection. He says that before he started using propranolol 1 year ago, he and his wife were sexually active without difficulties, but now he can achieve only a partial erection. He denies chest pain, palpitations, headaches, blackout spells, dyspnea, orthopnea, leg pain, weakness, paresthesias, or loss of muscle function. He admits to urinary hesitancy and nocturia.

Past Medical History

- 1960: Pneumonia—treated without sequelae.
- 1965: Pyelonephritis—treated without sequelae.
- 1990: Borderline hyperglycemia—Patient states he was told his glucose level was increased, but follow-up test results were "negative."
- 1991: Open-angle glaucoma—currently treated.
- Hospitalizations: 5 days in 1960 for repair of a right inguinal hernia.
- Surgery: Hernia repair in 1960, no problems.
- Drug allergies: None known.

Current Medications

- Propranolol: 40 mg orally twice a day
- Diltiazem: 60 mg orally three times a day
- Timolol: 0.25% 1 gtts twice a day
- Over-the-counter (OTC) ibuprofen: 200 mg orally three times a day as needed for joint pain

Family History

- Father died at 70 years of age from a myocardial infarction (MI).
- Mother is 90 years of age and "healthy as can be."
- Sister, 65 years of age, has type 2 diabetes mellitus (DM).
- Brother, 60 years of age, has hypertension and had an MI when he was 54 years of age.
- Son, 40 years of age, is healthy.
- Daughter, 35 years of age, is healthy.
- Wife, 72 years of age, is healthy.

The patient relates a family history of colon cancer in an uncle and an aunt (ages of diagnoses are unknown). He denies a family history of sickle cell disease, thalassemia, prostate cancer, or other familial disorders.

Social History

Patient is married and lives with his 72-year-old wife. He is a retired teacher, very active with his church, and an avid fisherman. He and his wife moved to this area to be closer to their grandchildren. He occasionally has a glass of wine but denies regular use of alcohol or tobacco. He denies a history of illicit drug use. He did smoke one pack of cigarettes each day from ages 18 to 41, then quit "cold turkey." He walks for 20 to 30 minutes two or three times each week with his wife.

Review of Systems

The patient describes his overall health as "fine" but has noticed dyspnea on exertion over the last 6 months, which he attributes to his age. He frequently has joint pain and stiffness in his fingers, especially at the end of the day. He treats this pain with regular use of OTC ibuprofen.

His medical records are incomplete, but upon review, you come across recent electrocardiogram (EKG) and chest x-ray reports that suggest cardiomegaly.

T A S K S

1. Develop a diagnoses list based on the patient's history.

2. What is the most likely cause of the complaint regarding difficulty in achieving full erection?

3. Should you be concerned that he is on propranolol and diltiazem?

4. Should you be concerned with his regular use of ibuprofen?

5. What is the most likely cause of the urinary hesitancy and nocturia?

6. What might the ophthalmoscopic examination reveal?

7. Regarding the family history, for what familial disorders should you screen him?

8. What is the most likely cause of his joint pain?

9. What findings on an EKG would suggest cardiomegaly?

10. What findings on a chest x-ray would suggest cardiomegaly?

11. What components of the physical examination (PE) would you emphasize?

12. What are the target organs of hypertension?

PHYSICAL EXAMINATION

General: Patient is a friendly and cooperative man of medium build who appears his stated age.

Vital signs: Pulse 55, regular; Respirations 16; Temperature 98.6°F (oral); Blood pressure 172/88 right arm/standing, 170/90 left arm/standing; Weight 170 lb; Height 5'10"; Osler maneuver indicates a palpable radial pulse when cuff pressure is raised above systolic blood pressure.

HEENT: Pupils equal, round, reactive to light and accommodation (PERRLA); arcus senilis bilaterally; visual fields intact; funduscopy reveals narrowing of arterioles, thickening and dulling of vessel reflection (copper-wire appearance); patent nares; oropharynx free of exudate, erythema, and lesions; noted upper dentures without lesions on gums

Neck: Supple without adenopathy, thyromegaly, or masses; trachea midline; carotids 2+ with right bruit, jugular venous distention (JVD)

Heart: Point of maximal impulse (PMI) in the fifth intercostal space (ICS) at the midclavicular line (MCL); regular rhythm with normal S1 and S2; S3 present; no murmurs or rubs

Chest: Symmetric expansion; resonant to percussion; clear to auscultation

Abdomen: Bowel sounds normoactive in all four quadrants; soft, non-tender; liver span 8 cm in the right MCL; no splenomegaly, masses, ascites, or bruits

Back: Spine midline without palpable masses or areas of tenderness; full range of motion (FROM) of the spine

Extremities: No cyanosis or clubbing; palpable peripheral pulses bilaterally equal; 1+ midtibial and pedal pitting edema bilaterally; no Heberden's or Bouchard's nodes on hands; minimal DIP/PIP bilateral joint hypertrophy with FROM and no tenderness

Genitourinary: Penis uncircumcised without masses or lesions; scrotum normal rugae without lesions; testes descended without masses; no hernia

Rectal: Nonthrombosed, nontender external hemorrhoid noted at the 12 o'clock position; no other external lesions; normal sphincter tone; prostate soft, smooth, nontender, unable to differentiate midline sulcus, palpable tip >1" in diameter; brown stool, guaiac negative

Neurologic: Cranial nerves II–VII intact; motor 5/5 upper and lower extremities; sensory intact to light/dull/sharp stimuli in upper and lower extremities; deep tendon reflexes (DTRs) 2+ and symmetric in the biceps, triceps, patellar, and Achilles' tendons

Mental status: Oriented to person, place, and time; appropriate affect, mood, and grooming

T A S K S

1. What are the abnormal PE findings? How are they significant?

2. Refine your list of diagnoses based on the information you now have.

3. Using the risk stratification criteria published by the National Institutes of Health in the Sixth Report of the Joint National Committee on Prevention, Detection, Evaluation, and Treatment of High Blood Pressure (JNC VI),[1] in what risk group and at what blood pressure stage is this patient?

4. What should his target blood pressure be?

5. What additional laboratory tests or diagnostic studies do you want to order?

6. Define what each study will contribute to your understanding of this patient.

7. Will Medicare pay for the studies you want?

8. What is Osler's maneuver?

LABORATORY TESTS AND DIAGNOSTIC STUDIES

There may be other initial or immediate laboratory tests or diagnostic studies that you could order at this time, but the following would form a basis for diagnosis and future monitoring.

1. Urinalysis (UA): Specific gravity is 1.025. Results are negative for blood, ketones, glucose, bilirubin, and leukocyte esterase. Protein is 1+. Microscopic results are negative for white blood cells (WBCs), red blood cells (RBCs), bacteria, and casts.
2. Electrolyte levels are as follows: sodium 130 mEq/L; potassium 4.5 mEq/L; chloride 101 mEq/L; carbon dioxide 22 mEq/L; fasting glucose 110 mg/dL; total calcium 7.0 mg/dL; magnesium 2.5 mEq/L; phosphorous 2.8 mg/dL; blood urea nitrogen (BUN) 30 mg/dL; creatinine 3.0 mg/dL.
3. Liver function test shows the following results: AST 40 U/L; ALT 35 U/L; alkaline phosphatase 180 U/L; total bilirubin 1.0 mg/dL; albumin 2.0 g/dL.
4. Complete blood count (CBC) is as follows: WBC 8,000/cu mm; hemoglobin 13.0 mg/dL; hematocrit 36%; platelets 350,000/cu mm; mean corpuscular volume (MCV) 87 fL; RDW 16.0.
5. New chest x-rays (Fig. 6–1) show mild cardiomegaly, normal mediastinum, and clear lungs.
6. New EKG results (Fig. 6–2) are as follows: sinus bradycardia at 54/min; QRS and ST-T wave changes suggestive of left ventricular hypertrophy; no Q waves; no axis deviation.

T A S K S

1. What is the significance of the abnormal results of the laboratory and diagnostic studies?

2. What is the significance of each of the following?
   A. Proteinuria: Does the patient have early nephropathy? What do you do to evaluate this?
   B. Borderline fasting glucose: Does he have diabetes? What additional testing would help you decide?

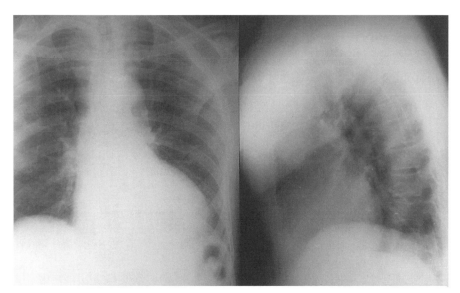

FIGURE 6–1   Chest x-ray of 70-year-old man with long-standing hypertension.

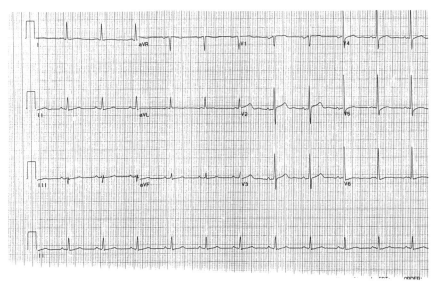

FIGURE 6–2   EKG of 70-year-old man with long-standing hypertension.

T A S K S (continued)

C. Elevated BUN and creatinine: What do these indicate? What further investigations should you do?
D. Cardiomegaly on chest x-ray: Does he have congestive heart failure (CHF)? Does his bradycardia contribute to his CHF, or is CHF the cause of his bradycardia?
E. Medications: What effects do his medications have on his complaints?

T A S K S

1. Considering the subjective and objective findings, what is your final diagnoses list?

2. What additional medical interventions should you consider at this time? Develop a medication regimen for Mr. Collier.

3. What other laboratory or diagnostic studies may now be indicated? For each one, describe what the test will tell you and how it will help you in the treatment of Mr. Collier. *Author's Note:* I suggest the following tests. Other studies may be needed, but those listed here would form a basis for diagnosis and future monitoring.
   A. Thyrotropin
   B. Sedimentation rate
   C. Lipid profile
   D. Prostate specific antigen
   E. Intraocular pressure testing/ophthalmologic referral
   F. Colonoscopy
   G. 24-hour protein/creatinine clearance collection
   H. Echocardiogram
   I. Guaiac cards for home use and return
   J. Glucose tolerance test
   K. Hemoglobin A_{1c}
   L. Carotid Doppler studies
   M. Local testing and documentation of blood pressure prior to follow-up appointment

POSSIBLE DIAGNOSES

There may be other diagnoses for this patient, but the following would form a basis from which to begin while the results of additional testing are pending.

- *Hypertension—essential:* The current regimen is not controlling the patient's blood pressure, and the use of propranolol may be contributing to the sinus bradycardia.
- *Renal impairment:* Proteinuria and elevated serum BUN and creatinine levels are possible signs of this condition.
- *Glaucoma:* This previous diagnosis warrants future monitoring.
- *Degenerative joint disease/osteoarthritis:* This condition is likely to be the diagnosis, based on history and PE findings, but it should be confirmed.
- *Erectile dysfunction:* This is most likely a side effect of propranolol, but organic or psychological causes should be investigated if needed.
- *Family history of colon cancer:* The appropriate screening should take place for this patient because of his family history.
- *Coronary artery disease (CAD):* This is based on the long-standing history of hypertension and the PE finding of a carotid bruit.
- *Possible early congestive heart failure:* This is the most likely cause of his symptoms of dyspnea on exertion, and it is supported by the PE finding. An echocardiogram should be ordered to confirm the diagnosis.
- *Benign prostatic hypertrophy (BPH):* This is most likely, based on the history and PE finding, but the appropriate screening for prostate cancer should be initiated.
- *Borderline hyperglycemia:* DM should be considered now and in the future because the patient is at an increased risk to develop this disorder. If he does not meet the diagnostic criteria for type 2 DM, he should be monitored in the future for its development.

GENERAL DISCUSSION

The patient's antihypertensive regimen is adjusted to address the concerns of erectile dysfunction, isolated systolic hypertension, BPH, early renal impairment, and suspected CHF. The patient is encouraged to avoid regular use of nonsteroidal anti-inflammatory drugs (NSAIDs) and to consider acetaminophen-based products. Regular use of NSAIDs may aggravate early renal impairment. The importance of compliance with his treatment regimen must be emphasized to him and to his family members.

The patient is encouraged to follow up with colonoscopy, 24-hour urine collection, echocardiogram, and monitoring of blood pressure. He also is urged to return guaiac cards on the follow-up visit. The patient is encouraged to begin taking half an aspirin daily and to make appropriate dietary and lifestyle modifications.

Using the JNC VI criteria, the patient is in risk group C because of the following risk factors: age older than 60 years, male sex, family history, hypertensive retinopathy, and heart disease demonstrated by left ventricular hypertrophy. His blood pressure is at stages 2 and 3. According to the same criteria, the patient's ideal blood pressure should be less than 130/85 mm Hg.

The decision to use a diuretic, beta blocker, angiotensin-converting enzyme (ACE) inhibitor, alpha blocker, or calcium channel blocker involves many variables such as age, sex, race/ethnicity, and underlying medical conditions. In this particular case, when deciding what antihypertensive regimen is most suitable, the clinician must consider that the patient is of African-American descent, is elderly, has multiple major risk factors, and has target organ damage and clinical cardiovascular disease.

African-Americans have the highest rates of hypertension of any racial group and also have a high rate of associated complications, such as end-organ damage.[2] According to the JNC VI, the medications most likely to benefit this patient include diuretics and ACE inhibitors.[1,2] Beta blockers do not appear to work as well as diuretics do in African-Americans.[2] In patients who are elderly and have CHF, diuretics have been proven to be beneficial.[2] ACE inhibitors should be used with caution in this case because of the underlying renal impairment.[2]

T A S K

Obtain a copy of the most recent JNC report, commit its concepts to memory, and understand how to apply them.

REFERENCES

1. The Sixth Report of the Joint National Committee on Prevention, Detection, Evaluation, and Treatment of High Blood Pressure. Bethesda, MD: National Institutes of Health; November 1997, NIH Publication No. 98-4080. Available at: www.nhlbi.nih.gov/guidelines/hypertension/jncintro.htm.
2. Stephenson KS. Hypertension management: Incorporating the JNC-VI recommendations in clinical practice. *Physician Assistant.* 1999;23(5):32–33.

Resource Notes

List all the references you used for this case.

"I Feel Tired and Have This Itching."

SALAH AYACHI, PhD, PA-C

BACKGROUND

You work in a community health clinic.

PATIENT HISTORY

A. Cuevas is a 59-year-old Hispanic homemaker and the mother of six children, ages 20 to 35 years. She was married to the same man for 35 years before his death from complications of alcohol-induced liver cirrhosis. Mrs. Cuevas has never used recreational drugs but did often drink at her late spouse's insistence. Although she misses her husband, she feels "liberated" and enjoys making independent decisions. Lately, Mrs. Cuevas has been experiencing fatigue, occasional dizziness, blurred vision, polyuria, and nocturia, all of which she attributes, at least in part, to "old age" and working to keep house for the two children who still live with her. In the past month, she has lost 15 lb but is trying to diet.

T A S K S

1. What additional history would you obtain from Mrs. Cuevas?

2. What clinical conditions could cause her symptoms?

3. For what diseases are Hispanics at high risk?

4. What are the social implications of adult children who still live at home?

5. What are the risk factors to consider when assessing this patient's problem?

ADDITIONAL HISTORY

Mrs. Cuevas considers herself relatively healthy, despite her recent concerns. She seldom complains; after all, she has the children to keep house for and feed. She denies any significant past health problems, and her review of systems (ROS) is noncontributory. She denies complications with the deliveries of her six children, all of which were spontaneous vaginal deliveries (SVDs) at the local hospital. She does not know if she had any pregnancy-induced problems. Mrs. Cuevas denies any psychiatric problems. She admits that she frequently argued with her late spouse about his drinking and "bad disposition" when drunk. Except for minor cuts secondary to culinary activities over the years, she denies significant trauma. She also denies hospitalizations other than stays for childbirth.

The patient is still active around the house, cooking for her two children and washing and ironing their clothing. She prepares three daily meals that include many starchy components. She enjoys *pan de dulce* every morning with coffee. She takes aspirin for occasional headaches and drinks an occasional beer but uses no tobacco or illicit drugs.

Mrs. Cuevas does not recall any details of her family history. Over the years, she has made only a few friends. She has devoted her life to her spouse and children. She is a devoutly religious person who derives strength from her faith.

Except for having to go to the bathroom at night and the increasingly bothersome itching that she has attempted to manage with skin lotion, she denies other problems. She has been 30 to 40 lb overweight most of her adult life.

She experienced menopause at age 50. She did not want hormone replacement therapy (HRT) because she did not want to menstruate.

T A S K S

1. From the history, develop a list of differential diagnoses.

2. What organ systems should you focus on in the physical examination (PE)?

3. List all the causes you can for unexplained weight loss.

4. How do you account for the patient's vision change?

5. How will you counsel her about HRT?

6. What nonmedical issues do you need to address with this patient?

PHYSICAL EXAMINATION

General: The patient, a mild-mannered Hispanic woman, looks overweight for her height.

Vital signs: Pulse 85, regular and bounding; Respirations 14; Temperature 99°F (oral); Blood pressure 150/90; Weight 161 lb; Height 5'1"

Skin: Several moles on neck and torso; skin in breast folds moist and macerated with a well-demarcated, bilateral, maculopapular erythemic rash

HEENT: Normocephalic; atraumatic; pupils equal, round, reactive to light and accommodation (PERRLA); arcus senilis present bilaterally; extraocular movements intact (EOMI); conjunctiva clear; pterygium extending from medial canthus halfway to limbus bilaterally; optic disc flat; no exudate or hemorrhages; mild arteriovenous (AV) nicking; Weber lateralizes to right; Rinne AC>BC

Mouth/pharynx: No lesions but missing several teeth; neck supple and with adenopathy; thyroid palpable on left side

Chest: Clear to auscultation; heart sounds normal; no murmurs, gallops, or rubs

Abdomen: Obese; bowel sounds active in all four quadrants, nontender; no hernias; striae present

Extremities: No clubbing or edema; toes cool to touch, with reddish-purple color involving toes and ankles; skin from midtibias down scaly and brownish; dorsalis pedis (DP) and posterior tibia (PT) pulses are 1+ bilaterally; capillary refill 3 seconds; patches of dilated veins in posterior aspects of thighs bilaterally

Musculoskeletal: Full range of motion (FROM) in all joints; slight tenderness in right knee; no edema, erythema, or effusion

Perineal area: Labia minor slightly erythemic; scant white discharge at introitus

Neurologic: AOX3; responses to questions appropriate; able to perform gaits; reflexes 2+ bilaterally at biceps, triceps, brachioradialis, patellar, and

Achilles; vibratory sense decreased bilaterally at metatarsal-phalangeal joints; decreased sharp and dull and fine touch senses below the ankles bilaterally; cranial nerves III–XII grossly intact

T A S K S

1. Based on the information you have, refine your list of diagnoses.

2. List the abnormalities found during the PE, and identify possible causes for each.

3. What laboratory studies and diagnostic tests would you like to obtain?

LABORATORY TESTS AND DIAGNOSTIC STUDIES

1. Random serum glucose value is 238 mg/dL.
2. Urinalysis (UA) dipstick shows glucose is 2+ and protein is 1+.
3. Glycosated hemoglobin (HbA_{1c}) is 8.2%.
4. Chest x-ray shows no cardiomegaly.
5. Electrocardiogram (EKG) shows normal sinus rhythm.
6. Complete blood count (CBC) results are as follows: white blood cells (WBCs) 4.2%; hemoglobin 12.5 g/dL; hematocrit 39.0%; platelets 158,000/cu mm.
7. Thyrotropin result is 0.8 mU/mL.

T A S K S

1. Refine your list of diagnoses based on the history, PE, and results of the laboratory tests and diagnostic studies.

2. What clues would support your diagnoses?

3. What additional studies should you order to further refine your list of final diagnoses?

4. Should you test for urine catecholamines?

5. Should you do a dexamethasone suppression test?

6. Is the HbA_{1c} level necessary to establish the diagnosis?

7. What tests could help identify the cause of her rash?

8. Should she have lipid studies, additional EKGs, liver function studies, or an eye examination?

9. What are the current criteria for establishing a diagnosis of diabetes mellitus (DM)?

10. What clinical clues would lead you to consider type 2 versus type 1 DM?

11. How would you treat this patient (medication, lifestyle changes, diet, exercise, home monitoring)?

12. What medications would you select for this patient considering her other coexisting problems?

GENERAL DISCUSSION

The primary diagnosis for this patient is type 2 DM. Secondary diagnoses include hypertension, dermal candidiasis, and obesity. Type 2 DM affects nearly 6% of the U. S. population, with African-Americans, Hispanics, and Native-Americans being affected in higher proportions than white Americans. Similarly, patients with first-degree relatives who have DM have an increased incidence of this disease. Uncontrolled DM results in serious complications, all of which are attributable to microvascular and macrovascular damage.

Mrs. Cuevas presents with some classic manifestations of type 2 DM: polyuria, nocturia, fatigue, weight loss, and vision change. She has two risk factors—Hispanic ethnicity and obesity—that definitely increase her chance of developing DM. An associated sign is fungal infection of the skin under the breasts, which can be attributed to *Candida*. The blood glucose level drawn during her visit to your clinic is above 200 mg/dL, and in itself is a diagnostic criterion. The HbA_{1c} level, not recommended for diagnosis, is above normal. The decrease in vibratory and sharp/dull sensations in the feet and the decrease in the peripheral pulses is consistent with complications of DM.

Mrs. Cuevas needs further evaluation for hypertension and hyperlipidemia, both of which often coexist with and further aggravate the vascular complications of DM, particularly in the kidneys and retinas. Evidence of early renal damage appears in the UA, which shows proteinuria; the glucosuria is expected given the blood glucose levels. She also needs a dilated funduscopic examination by an ophthalmologist.

Management of this patient's condition may or may not be difficult depending on many factors, including her general attitude and outlook on life and willingness to engage in novel activities. This patient has generally devoted herself to family and family needs; she still attends to her grown children. As a health-care professional, you are faced with the challenge of educating this patient to make the lifestyle changes necessary to impact the disease process. You would do well to involve her children in her care by teaching them how to regularly inspect her feet, how to encourage adherence to prescribed exercise regimens, how to assist their mother in home monitoring of glucose, and how to monitor her compliance with medications. You should also engage a social worker to identify community resources for transportation, support groups, exercise, and weight loss.

The cornerstones of therapy for patients with type 2 DM are diet and exercise. Exercise enhances the patient's sense of well-being, improves glucose metabolism, and reduces tissue resistance to insulin.[1] Exercise also reduces blood pressure, helps reduce body weight, and ameliorates dyslipidemia.

In this case, treatment with an oral hypoglycemic agent such as metformin (Glucophage) should be instituted without delay, in anticipation of some reticence on the patient's part. A renal-sparing antihypertensive agent such as lisinopril or other angiotensin-converting enzyme (ACE) inhibitor may be used to control blood pressure.[1] Beta blockers and thiazides should be avoided because of their untoward effects on β-cell function and the possibility of blocking hypoglycemic symptoms. Treatment of candidiasis of the skin requires a topical antifungal agent such as clotrimazole 1% applied twice daily for 10 to 14 days. Vaginal candidiasis would require management using any one of several different local or systemic regimens. Referral of the patient to an ophthalmologist for screening and evaluation of diabetic retinopathy is necessary.

Successful management of DM calls for regular follow-up at 4-week intervals (some providers may differ with this schedule) until her glycemia is controlled, then monitoring every 3 to 4 months.[2] During these visits, focus should be on glycemic control, reinforcement of diet and exercise regimens, encouragement of patient adherence, and psychological support of the patient. Control of DM as well as treatment of hypertension should be individualized and approached in stepwise fashion.[1]

T A S K S

1. Learn to do finger sticks for glucose. Then practice teaching the patient how to do them.

2. How often should the patient check her glucose as part of home monitoring?

3. How much does metformin cost?

4. Should you have asked the patient about her sexual activities (if you didn't)?

5. What is the formula for calculating insulin dose?

6. What are the indications for insulin need in patients with DM?

7. What are the types of insulin?

8. How do you choose a type of insulin for a patient?

9. Learn to educate a patient about a diabetic diet.

10. What are the complications of uncontrolled DM?

REFERENCES

1. Lipsky MS. Type II diabetes. In Rakel RE, ed. *Essentials of Family Practice*. 2nd ed. Philadelphia: WB Saunders; 1998:457–463.
2. Gray DS. Diabetes mellitus, Type 2. In Dambro MR, ed. *Griffith's 5-Minute Clinical Consult 2000*. Philadelphia: Lippincott Williams & Wilkins; 2000:314–315.

Resource Notes

List all the references you used for this case.

CASE 8

"I Think I Have AIDS."

ROBERTO CANALES, MS, PA-C

BACKGROUND

You work in an outpatient human immunodeficiency virus (HIV) clinic in an academic health science center.

PATIENT HISTORY

Brenda Sue Doe is a 37-year-old woman who presents for initial evaluation of HIV infection. Ten months ago, a relative informed her of the death of Ms. Doe's ex-husband from complications of acquired immunodeficiency syndrome (AIDS). Ms. Doe waited 4 months to get tested anonymously, and the result was positive for HIV infection.

Ms. Doe has not seen anyone for this condition and adds that it has taken her this long to build up the courage to make an appointment. During the past 12 months, she has experienced four episodes of vaginal candidiasis in addition to malaise, fatigue, and swollen neck glands. Before these developments, she had been healthy. She currently denies weight loss, fevers, night sweats, diarrhea, or cough.

T A S K S

1. What should the diagnoses list consist of at this point?

2. What additional history do you want?

3. In what stage of HIV might the patient be?

4. What might the absolute CD4 count be?

5. What might the HIV quantifiable viral load be?

6. Other than HIV infection, what other illnesses might be contributing to or causing her symptoms?

7. Identify all the ways that a person can contract or transmit HIV infection.

ADDITIONAL HISTORY

Ms. Doe self-diagnosed and treated each episode of presumed vaginal candidiasis with over-the-counter (OTC) medication and is currently without vaginal complaints. Her menstrual cycles are regular, and her last menstrual period (LMP) ended 2 weeks ago.

During the last 3 months, malaise and fatigue have increased and now interfere with her ability to complete household chores and care for her 8-year-old and 10-year-old sons. Also, she has noticed tenderness of the lymph nodes in her neck but nowhere else. She adds that foods do not taste the same, and 2 days ago she developed a sore throat.

She denies additional risk factors for HIV infection, such as blood transfusions. She denies a history of tuberculosis (TB) exposure, hepatitis, sexually transmitted diseases (STDs), substance abuse, and surgical procedures. Her family history is unremarkable, and she currently denies alcohol or tobacco use. The general review of symptoms (ROS) is unremarkable for changes in the skin, headaches, shortness of breath, or easy bruising.

Ms. Doe divorced her ex-husband 2 years ago, ending a 10-year marriage. He moved to another state, and she did not stay in contact with him nor did he attempt to visit their children. Ms. Doe initiated the divorce after experiencing years of verbal abuse by her ex-husband. She adds that this abuse was associated with his use of cocaine and alcohol. She knew he was sexually promiscuous but never thought she would contract HIV infection.

For fear of repercussions, she has told no one in her family (including her sons) about her HIV status nor has she told her employer. She is a third-grade teacher in the local public school system.

Ms. Doe does not have a current sexual partner but was involved in a 2-month relationship with a male colleague that ended when she became aware of her HIV status. During this relationship, she and this man were sexually active, and they did not use barrier protection. She has not informed him of the HIV test result. She fears discrimination in the community and workplace for herself and her former partner if this information becomes known.

She relates that her sons are having behavioral difficulties in school related to the divorce and death of their father. The children were told that their father died of cancer.

She has tried to remain optimistic by going to church every Sunday and praying for her family's welfare, but the stress of keeping her HIV infection a secret is becoming overwhelming. During the last few weeks, she has experienced difficulty falling asleep, often lying in bed for hours. She begins to cry for no apparent reason but goes on "for my kids." She states that because of her strong religious faith and love for her children, suicide has never crossed her mind. She denies recent weight gain, weight loss, and pregnancy.

T A S K S

1. Has this additional information affected your list of potential diagnoses?

2. What is the HIV partner notification policy in your community?

3. Has the additional information changed your expectations of values for the absolute CD4 count and the HIV quantifiable viral load?

4. What is the difference (if any) between having HIV infection and having AIDS?

5. According to the HIV classification system of the Centers for Disease Control and Prevention (CDC), what are the diagnostic criteria for AIDS?

6. What are the key components to focus on in the physical examination (PE)?

PHYSICAL EXAMINATION

General: Patient is an alert, cooperative, well-groomed woman. She appears slightly anxious and older than stated age. She is oriented × 3, in no acute distress, and not crying.

Vital signs: Pulse 78, regular; Respirations 16, unlabored; Temperature 99.8°F (oral); Blood pressure 128/84, right arm, sitting; Weight 130 lb; Height 5′6″

Skin: Warm and dry with normal texture and turgor; no lesions or rashes

Head: Normocephalic, atraumatic; appropriate distribution of hair without lesions; face symmetrical; nontender to palpation

Eyes: By handheld chart visual acuity 20/20 OU without glasses; visual fields intact to confrontation; conjunctiva pink; sclera anicteric; cornea without opacities; extraocular movements intact (EOMI); pupils equal, round, reactive to light and accommodation (PERRLA); no lid lag or nystagmus

Funduscopic: Red reflex present; sharp disc margins; no exudates, hemorrhages, or arteriovenous (AV) nicking

Ears: External auditory canals (EACs) patent without erythema, edema, or exudate; tympanic membranes (TMs) mobile and pearly grey with visible landmarks and cone of light; hearing acuity intact to whisper; Weber midline; Rinne AC>BC

Nose: Septum midline; mucosa pink without bogginess, discharge, drainage, or polyps; nares patent; sinuses nontender

Mouth: Good dentition with few fillings; mucosa with bilateral diffuse white plaques laterally, otherwise without lesions; hard and soft palate intact; tonsils present, without erythema or exudate; uvula midline

Neck: Full range of motion (FROM); trachea midline; thyroid nonpalpable; no bruits or jugular venous distention (JVD)

Chest: Symmetrical with normal spinal curvature; nontender to palpation; diaphragmatic excursion 3 cm on right and 4 cm on left; symmetrical expansion; resonant to percussion; clear to auscultation without adventitious sounds bilaterally; tactile fremitus normal

Breasts: Equal in size and shape; skin without lesions; no masses or nipple discharge

Heart: Quiet precordium; point of maximal impulse (PMI) at fifth intercostal space (ICS) of midclavicular line (MCL); regular rate and rhythm with normal S1 and S2; no murmurs, rubs, or gallops; no lifts, heaves, or thrills

Abdomen: Flat without striae; normoactive bowel sounds throughout without bruits; nontender to light palpation but some guarding on deep palpation of right upper quadrant; no rebound tenderness or guarding; liver percussed at 10 cm right MCL; kidneys and spleen not palpable; no masses or costovertebral angle tenderness; noted suprapubic transverse scar tissue

Genitourinary: External genitalia normal without lesions, swelling, or discharge; vagina pink with normal rugae; noted two 2- $\times$ 2-mm cauliflower lesions on internal vaginal wall at the 1 and 2 o'clock positions; cervix pink without lesions or discharge; uterus midline, anterior, smooth, not enlarged; adnexa palpable, mobile, nontender, without enlargement or masses; cervix mobile and nontender

Rectal: No visible masses or lesions; normal sphincter tone; no palpable masses; hemoccult test negative

Lymph: Bilateral, pea-size-deep cervical chain nodes, nontender, soft, mobile; otherwise, no axillary or inguinal nodes palpable

Extremities: No clubbing, cyanosis, edema, lesions, or scars; FROM; strength 5 bilaterally over all major muscles

Neurologic/vascular: Cranial nerves I–XII grossly intact; pronation/supination, point to point intact; Romberg, Babinski, and clonus negative; gait intact; light touch, sharp/dull, vibratory, and stereognosis intact

Reflexes	Biceps	Triceps	Brachioradialis	Patellar	Achilles
Right	2+	2+	2+	2+	2+
Left	2+	2+	2+	2+	2+

2+ = normal

Pulses	Radial	Femoral	Popliteal	Dorsalis Pedis (DP)	Posterior Tibia (PT)
Right	4+	4+	4+	4+	4+
Left	4+	4+	4+	4+	4+

4+ = normal

T A S K S

1. What were the abnormal PE findings?

2. How have the abnormal PE findings affected your diagnoses list?

3. As a result of the abnormal PE findings, what additional subjective information would you obtain at this time?

FURTHER HISTORY BASED ON PE FINDINGS

Ms. Doe states that she has noticed a thick white plaque inside her mouth for the last 2 days and adds that she can brush it off with her toothbrush. She also has noticed the cervical chain nodes and adds that, although they are not tender now, they have been in the past. She denies a history of genital condyloma but adds, "With everything he gave me, I wouldn't be surprised if he gave me that also." Her last Papanicolaou test was 2 years ago, and the result was "normal."

T A S K S

---

1. Develop and refine your diagnoses list for this patient.

2. What laboratory or diagnostic studies would you order at this time?

3. Justify each of your choices by explaining how the results will help you in your evaluation, treatment, and monitoring of this patient.

POSSIBLE DIAGNOSES

There may be other diagnoses for this patient, but the following would form a basis from which to begin while the results of additional testing are pending:

- HIV infection by history
- Multiple situational stressors
- Oral candidiasis
- Hepatomegaly (assess for viral hepatitis)
- Vaginal condyloma acuminata
- Recurrent presumed vaginal candidiasis
- Situational depression
- Partner notification required

POSSIBLE DIAGNOSTIC STUDIES

There may be other laboratory tests or diagnostic studies that would be needed, but the following would form a basis for diagnosis and future monitoring:

- HIV test—to confirm HIV infection
- Complete blood count (CBC) with differential—to assess for anemia of chronic disease and for baseline purposes prior to antiretroviral therapy
- CD4 lymphocyte panel—to assess for the risk of opportunistic infection; because of findings consistent with oral candidiasis, the absolute CD4 count is likely to be no greater than 400 mm^3
- HIV quantifiable viral load—to assess for the risk of disease progression; because of the patient's signs and symptoms, the HIV viral load is likely to be greater than 20,000 copies/mL
- Electrolytes—mainly for baseline purposes

- Rapid plasma reagin (RPR)—because of the risk of becoming infected with syphilis in conjunction with HIV
- Liver function test—to assess for baseline purposes prior to antiretroviral therapy and because of hepatomegaly on PE
- Immunoglobulin G (IgG) for toxoplasmosis and cytomegalovirus—to assess for prior infection to determine the risk for reactivation should the absolute CD4 count drop below 100 mm³
- Hepatitis panel—because of the risk of becoming infected with hepatitis B, hepatitis C, or both in conjunction with HIV
- Chest x-ray—considered for baseline purposes
- Urinalysis (UA)—to assess for proteinuria, which may be an early indication of HIV-associated nephropathy

T A S K S

1. What medical interventions should you consider at this time?

2. Consider the value of each of the following, and discuss what they mean to your patient.
A. Beck inventory (or similar) instrument to evaluate for depression.
B. Social service consult.
C. The need to have the patient or the local health department notify the previous sexual partner of his exposure to HIV (a documented HIV test from your institution should be obtained first).
D. A gynecology referral for treatment of the presumed vaginal condyloma and for a Papanicolaou test to assess for dysplasia. A routine Papanicolaou test should be performed every 6 to 12 months, unless findings warrant more frequent testing or treatment.
E. Patient education regarding HIV.
F. Tuberculin skin test.
G. Pneumococcal vaccine.
H. Influenza vaccine (if appropriate).
I. Referral or access to an available community support agency.

3. What medical interventions would you prescribe at this time?

4. What current antiretroviral recommendations are appropriate for Ms. Doe if her HIV test is positive?

5. What about antidepressants?

6. When should Ms. Doe return for the follow-up appointment?

ADDITIONAL DATA

The patient reports for follow-up 3 weeks later and says that the oral symptoms have resolved and that the diphenhydramine helped her fall asleep. The tender cervical lymph nodes have persisted along with the malaise and fatigue. On four separate occasions, she experienced drenching night sweats without fever or weight loss. She denies alcohol or drug use.

She met with her ex-boyfriend the day after the initial visit, and he had an HIV test performed anonymously. His initial test result came back negative, but he will take another test in a few months. He has agreed to keep this information confidential. She has decided not to tell her children and would like to work as long as possible. She is also anxious to begin antiretroviral therapy.

LABORATORY TESTS AND DIAGNOSTIC STUDIES

1. The results of the enzyme-linked immunosorbent assay (ELISA) and Western blot tests for HIV are both positive.
2. Absolute CD4 count is 220 mm^3.
3. Polymerase chain reaction (PCR) HIV viral load is 40,000 copies/mL.
4. Results of liver function tests are as follows: AST 120 U/L; ALT 160 U/L; alkaline phosphatase 200 U/L; total bilirubin 1.0 mg/dL; albumin 2.0 g/dL; GGTP 170.
5. Hepatitis panel shows the following results: negative for hepatitis BsAg and BcAb and IgM/IgG; positive for hepatitis C Ab.
6. Additional test results, including the purified protein derivative (PPD), were essentially unremarkable or negative.

T A S K S

1. How do these laboratory results affect your staging of Ms. Doe's HIV infection and your diagnoses list?

2. What antiretroviral combination therapy would you prescribe at this time? (*Author's Note:* The decision not to initiate antiretroviral therapy in someone with a normal CD4 lymphocyte count and no quantifiable virus in the plasma using ultrasensitive testing should be considered.[1] Most authorities use viral loads >5000 copies/mL of plasma and a normal or decreased absolute CD4 count as an indicator to initiate therapy.[1] For initial therapy in an individual who is treatment-naive, common practice is to combine one protease inhibitor (PI) with two nucleoside reverse transcriptase inhibitors (NRTIs) or two NRTIs with one non-nucleoside reverse transcriptase inhibitor (NNRTI).[1] Alternative therapies include a multitude of antiretrovirals or a combination of PIs, NRTIs, and NNRTIs.)

3. Would you prescribe additional medications for prophylaxis of certain opportunistic infections? (*Author's Note:* Despite a CD4 lymphocyte count above 200 mm^3, Bactrim DS should be considered as prophylaxis for pneumocystis pneumonia. Many variables can influence the CD4 lymphocyte count, such as the time of day, time of year, laboratory performing the test, or intercurrent infection. The diurnal variation in CD4 counts averages 60 mm^3 higher in the afternoon in those with HIV infection.[1] For this reason, Bactrim DS once a day Monday through Friday should be initiated for prophylaxis. Alternative medications can be used.)

4. Would you consider referring Ms. Doe to a gastroenterologist/ hepatologist? If so, why and for what purpose? (*Author's Note:* Ms. Doe is anti-HCV antibody positive and has elevated liver enzyme levels. For this reason, referral to a gastroenterologist or hepatologist should be placed for further evaluation and possible treatment. Antiviral drugs such as interferon can be used alone or in combination with ribavirin for the treatment of persons with chronic hepatitis C.[2])

5. When should she return to the clinic? (*Author's Note:* Routinely, a 1-month follow-up should take place when antiretroviral therapy is being instituted to assess for adverse drug reactions, side effects, compliance, and response to therapy.)

GENERAL DISCUSSION

Infection with HIV continues to spread, inflicting pain and suffering not only on individuals but also on partners, spouses, and extended families. A recent analysis suggested that, despite a declining trend in AIDS diagnoses, newly reported HIV cases continue to disproportionately affect women and minorities. From July 1998 through June 1999, a total of 47,083 AIDS cases were reported.[3] Women accounted for 10,841 (23%) of the reported cases. Among women, African-Americans and Hispanics accounted for 80% of cases.[3]

Women accounted for 32% of adult cases of HIV infection reported from July 1998 through June 1999.[3] Among women, African-Americans and Hispanics accounted for 77% of cases. Persons 13 to 24 years of age accounted for 15% of reported HIV cases, and women accounted for 49% of cases in this age group.[3]

Risk information is not always readily available. For this reason, a practitioner should not develop "tunnel vision" when trying to determine if an HIV test is warranted. Most sexually active adults have some degree of risk of becoming infected with HIV regardless of identifiable risk factors and should be offered an HIV test.

REFERENCES

1. Sande AM, Gilbert ND, Moelering CR. *The Sanford Guide to HIV/AIDS Therapy.* 8th ed. Vermont: Antimicrobial Therapy Inc; 1999:9–15.
2. Centers for Disease Control and Prevention. Viral Hepatitis C—Frequently Asked Questions. Available at: http://www.cdc.gov/ncidod/diseases/hepatitis/c/faq.htm
3. Centers for Disease Control and Prevention. HIV/AIDS Surveillance Report. U.S. HIV and AIDS cases reported through June 1999. Midyear edition Vol. 11, No. 1. Available at: http://www.cdc.gov/hiv/stats/hasrlink.htm

Resource Notes

List all the references you used for this case.

"My Chest Hurts!"

SALAH AYACHI, PhD, PA-C

BACKGROUND

You are working in a small-town hospital, covering the inpatients for a group of family physicians.

PATIENT HISTORY

C. Diaz, a 55-year-old Hispanic man, is a "down-on-his-luck" Vietnam veteran. Twice divorced, he is the father of three children whose whereabouts are unknown. He is currently unemployed and living on meager benefits. Mr. Diaz has a long history of alcohol use (one to two six-packs of beer each day for the last 15 years) and tobacco smoking (two packs of cigarettes each day for the last 30 years). He also has "dabbled" in illicit drugs but has never "injected." He has been involved in a few altercations while drunk, resulting in a broken nose and lacerations that healed without difficulty.

His only sister brings Mr. Diaz to the emergency department (ED). He complains of dyspnea and mild substernal pain. He denies diaphoresis, nausea, vomiting, hemoptysis, or hematemesis. While helping his sister with chores around the house, he noticed the pain, which he ignored until he became short of breath (SOB). She insisted that he seek medical attention. He admits to a similar episode 3 to 4 months ago, which he ignored. He attributes the dyspnea to being overweight, smoking cigarettes, and "not taking care of myself." His sister comments, "Charley has never been the same since the war. I try to help him whenever I can, but life is tough on everyone. He won't go to the VA."

T A S K S

1. What other history questions would you like to ask the patient?

2. What clinical conditions should you consider based on the information you have obtained?

3. What are possible causes of this patient's chest pain?

4. What cardiac and other risk factors should you consider in evaluating this patient?

5. What is the significance of his two divorces and the fact that he has no contact with his children? Would this affect his treatment and possible outcomes?

ADDITIONAL HISTORY

Mr. Diaz considers his health to be "OK," even though he eats fatty foods, smokes, drinks, and does not exercise. He considers himself "lucky so far" except for a bout of pneumonia in 1987, when he woke up "choking on saliva." He denies psychiatric problems, even though he admits to coping with argumentative wives, being unable to keep a job, and having a bad disposition when inebriated. His sister reports, "Someone broke his nose several years ago in a bar fight. He also fell and broke his right ankle one evening returning from a bar. He thinks he has hardware in his right ankle. I think his memory is going bad."

Mr. Diaz is not very active physically, although he has much free time. He does odd jobs for money. Meals are irregular and often heavy on fats and starches. He enjoys donuts and coffee when he wakes up.

He refuses to discuss his family history and becomes belligerent when his sister wants to say something about it. He has no living friends. He cannot tell whether he has polyuria or polydipsia because of his drinking.

T A S K S

1. What body systems should you focus on in the physical examination (PE)?

2. What other systems should you include in your work-up?

3. List every physical, mental, and social risk factor you can identify for this patient.

4. Given the history and the risk factors, what would you expect to find on the PE?

PHYSICAL EXAMINATION

General: Patient appears uncomfortable. He denies current pain.

Vital signs: Pulse 75, regular and bounding; Respirations 18; Temperature 98.4°F (oral); Blood pressure 160/90; Weight 285 lb; Height 5′ 8″

HEENT: Normocephalic; hair gray and thin; nasal septum deviated to right side; pupils equal, round, reactive to light and accommodation (PERRLA); extraocular movements intact (EOMI); conjunctiva clear; optic discs flat; no exudate or hemorrhages; mild arteriovenous (AV) nicking; Weber midline; Rinne AC>BC

Mouth/pharynx: No lesions; nearly edentulous (four upper teeth, eight lower teeth, all with plaque or caries); tongue green with tobacco stain

Neck: Supple and without adenopathy; thyroid nonpalpable; jugular venous distention (JVD) to 5 cm

Chest/lungs: Percussion resonant to slightly hyperresonant; tactile fremitus decreased; expiratory wheezing and coarse rhonchi in both bases; diaphragmatic excursion 3 cm bilaterally

Heart: Normal S1 and S2 with no murmurs, gallops, or rubs; point of maximal impulse (PMI) displaced to the left

Abdomen: Obese; bowel sounds active in all four quadrants, nontender; no hernias; striae present; liver span 14 cm at midclavicular line (MCL); no splenomegaly

Extremities: Early clubbing; toes cool to touch; nails thick, yellow, and brittle; scaling, red skin in web spaces of both feet; trace pretibial edema; skin from midtibias down scaly and brownish; dorsalis pedis (DP) and posterior tibia (PT) pulses are 1+ bilaterally; capillary refill 3 seconds

Musculoskeletal: Full range of motion (FROM) in all joints; no edema, except as noted above; no erythema or effusion; no tenderness of costochondral joints; no rib tenderness

Neurologic: AOX3; responses to questions appropriate; able to perform gaits; reflexes 2+ bilaterally at biceps, triceps, brachioradialis, patellar, and

Achilles; unable to identify vibratory sense at metatarsal-phalangeal joint of great toes, but intact at malleoli bilaterally; decreased sharp and dull and fine touch senses below the ankles bilaterally; cranial nerves III–XII grossly intact

T A S K S

1. What are your preliminary differential diagnoses based on the patient's history and PE?

2. What laboratory tests and diagnostic studies would be necessary to support, add to, or eliminate some of the differential diagnoses?

3. What priority would you give to each test?

4. While you are waiting for the tests you want to be done, what do you do for the patient (for example, start oxygen)?

LABORATORY TESTS AND DIAGNOSTIC STUDIES

1. A chest x-ray shows emphysematous changes and fluid meniscus in the left costophrenic space (gutter) on posteroanterior (PA) view. Heart is slightly enlarged.
2. Electrocardiogram (EKG) (Fig. 9–1) shows left ventricular hypertrophy, left atrial hypertrophy, nonspecific T-wave changes, and early repolarization. Serial EKGs do not change.
3. CK-MB at 2 and 6 hours postpresentation to ED are normal.
4. Liver function tests show elevated gamma-glutamyltransferase (GGT) (335 U/L); other enzymes only slightly elevated.
5. Lipase equals 650 U/L.
6. Random blood glucose is 273 mg/dL.

T A S K S

1. Use the history, PE, and laboratory and diagnostic studies to further redefine your diagnoses.

2. Does Mr. Diaz have an emergent, life-threatening condition? Do you have enough information to make that determination?

3. Would any additional studies help you evaluate this patient?

4. How would you prioritize the above studies to narrow your differential diagnoses?

5. Will a Holter monitor help?

6. Should you just send the patient home, telling him to take Motrin and prescribing a muscle relaxant for musculoskeletal pain?

7. Would you admit the patient for observation?

8. Should you start the patient on an oral hypoglycemic agent before he leaves the ED?

9. Why are the GGT and lipase levels so high?

10. Did the patient have a silent myocardial infarction (MI)?

11. Do you have enough information to say that he has not had an MI?

12. Should you order an upper gastrointestinal (GI) series? If so, why?

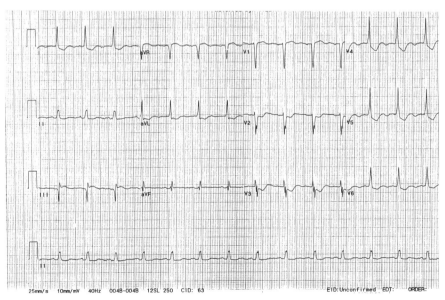

FIGURE 9–1   EKG on admission to ED.

13. Prioritize your diagnoses from most serious to least serious.

14. What problems do you address first and why?

15. Assess the probability of successful management of this patient.

16. What laboratory tests can be used to evaluate MI? What are their patterns and interpretations?

17. Each of the following problems causes chest pain. Discuss what you would do to evaluate, treat, and monitor:
A. MI
B. Angina pectoris
C. Gastroesophageal reflux disease (GERD)
D. Costochondritis
E. Pneumonia
F. Liver cirrhosis
G. Bleeding esophageal varices
H. Peptic ulcer disease
I. Pancreatitis
J. Psychosomatic pain

GENERAL DISCUSSION

The primary diagnosis for this patient is angina induced by physical exertion. Remember the classic definition of angina is pain on exertion relieved by rest, which his history matches. Secondary diagnoses include GERD, alcoholic liver disease, obesity, probable type 2 diabetes mellitus (DM), tobacco abuse, early emphysema, chronic pancreatitis, hypertension, depression, and post-traumatic stress disorder.

Mr. Diaz presents with classic manifestations of angina pectoris—pain brought on by exertion and relieved by rest. He has several risk factors: high dietary fat intake, hypertension, alcoholism, smoking, and Hispanic ethnicity. These same risk factors also predispose him to the development of type 2 DM. His blood pressure is high, and his random blood glucose drawn during his visit to the ED is above 200 mg/dL, in itself a diagnostic criterion for DM. He has a 45-year history of tobacco use and has drunk alcohol for many years. Given his mental status, Mr. Diaz is not likely to adhere to treatment regimens, which will make management of his many conditions rather difficult.

Mr. Diaz should be referred for counseling. A VA hospital, if possible, may be his best opportunity to effect changes in his outlook on life and to receive help in ending alcohol and tobacco use. Similarly, he needs help to access medical services either at the VA hospital itself or at a point-of-service on contract with the VA. This is very important for successful management of the patient. His sister could be included, whenever possible, in "redirecting" the patient; it appears Mr. Diaz has some affinity for his sister and would likely listen to her. Without psychological intervention, efforts to limit his dietary fats, to curtail his smoking and drinking of alcohol, and to control his DM may not be fruitful.

Nevertheless, the health-care professional should resolve to promote behavioral changes in Mr. Diaz that are conducive to the amelioration of the patient's condition(s). Mr. Diaz needs encouragement to attend Alcoholics Anonymous meetings and to set realistic goals and deadlines for reducing and eventually ceasing alcohol and tobacco use. He requires close monitoring and continual encouragement to pursue these goals.

Treatment of the angina may be with short-acting or long-acting nitroglycerin preparations (tablet, oral spray, or patch), beta blockers (for example, atenolol, metoprolol, nadolol), calcium channel blockers (for example, diltiazem, verapamil), and aspirin.

Management of DM can start with weight loss, abstinence from alcohol, and modification of dietary habits without an initial need for medications. If Mr. Diaz fails to implement these changes, he may be started on an oral hypoglycemic agent, with regular monitoring of his blood glucose, and dose titration to achieve euglycemia. Similarly, management of hypertension could be through weight loss, graded physical exercise, and abstinence from alcohol. If not, an angiotensin-converting enzyme (ACE) inhibitor (known for renal protective effects) may be introduced to control blood pressure, with the dosage titrated.

To determine disease progression, levels of pancreatic lipase (pancreatitis) and GGT (alcoholic hepatitis) require regular monitoring. Hb A_{1c} levels also must be measured at intervals to aid in determining the success of DM management. A stress test should be performed to assess the degree of coronary artery disease (CAD) and as a guide for further evaluation.

Mr. Diaz should be educated that patients with a history of hyperlipidemia who are overweight, have a strong family history of CAD and hypertension, smoke cigarettes, and have sedentary lifestyles are at high risk of sudden death.

T A S K S

> **1.** Practice your patient education skills by doing the following:
>   A. Helping the patient monitor his blood pressure and keep a log
>   B. Showing him how to do a finger stick to measure glucose at home and how to keep a log

2. Identify social services available in your community to which you could refer Mr. Diaz.

3. Should you inquire about the patient's sexual activities? If not, why not?

4. What are the complications of uncontrolled DM?

5. What are the complications of uncontrolled hypertension?

6. What are the complications of chronic pancreatitis?

7. What are the cutaneous manifestations of liver disease?

8. If Mr. Diaz does nothing, what is his prognosis? How would you handle his refusal to do anything to change his life?

9. Would you insist that the patient be tested for the human immunodeficiency virus (HIV)? What about tests for other sexually transmitted diseases (STDs)?

10. Think about and discuss the psychological and social components of this patient's problems.

SUGGESTED READINGS

Corboy JE. Chest pain. In Rakel RE, ed. *Essentials of Family Medicine.* 2nd ed. Philadelphia: WB Saunders; 1998:342–349.
Ferri FF. *Practical Guide to the Care of the Medical Patient.* 4th ed. St Louis: Mosby; 1998.

Resource Notes

List all the references you used for this case.

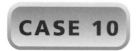

"I Hurt My Back!"

J. DENNIS BLESSING, PhD, PA-C

BACKGROUND

You work in a rural health clinic in a small community (population 1,500). Your supervising physician is 25 miles away in a larger community that has a 20-bed hospital.

PATIENT HISTORY

James Williams is a 45-year-old African-American who is the head of bus maintenance at the local elementary and middle school. Shortly after changing the tires on a school bus yesterday, he experienced the onset of low back pain, which continues to worsen. He has had previous back injuries. Mr. Williams has hypertension, which he currently controls with medication, and a strong family history of cardiovascular disease.

T A S K S

1. Review the anatomy of the back.

2. What should you ask as part of the history of the present illness?

3. Should you be concerned about a cardiologic or peripheral vascular cause of his back pain?

4. What other organ systems may manifest problems as back pain?

5. What does changing the tires on a school bus entail, and how big are the tires?

6. What is the incidence and morbidity of back pain and injury in the United States?

ADDITIONAL HISTORY

The patient has felt well and had no physical problems until the back pain began. He and another worker had changed all the tires, which were large, heavy, and bulky, on a big bus. Mr. Williams had a tough time removing the lug nuts, using a tire tool with an extension. He felt some pulling up and down his back while working, but it was not painful. He had no direct injury or trauma to his back. About 1 hour after changing the tire, he felt stiffness in his back with a mild (3 on a scale of 1 to 10) pain in his middle to lower back. He continued his routine work, which did not require exertion, the rest of the day. By last night, his back was stiff and painful (8 on a scale of 1 to 10). The pain was located in the "small of his back." He took two aspirins and drank a few beers, which relieved the pain slightly. He had difficulty sleeping during the night. This morning, he rates the pain as 8 on a scale of 1 to 10, and he also has pain in his right buttock. There is no other radiculopathy and no paresthesias, loss of sensation, or muscle weakness. He has no incontinence, blood in his urine, dysuria, or problems starting or stopping his urine stream. He has had no nausea, vomiting, or diarrhea. He has no chest pain, shortness of breath, or diaphoresis. He continues to take his prescribed medications, which consist of hydrochlorothiazide 25 mg once a day, amlodipine 10 mg once a day, and aspirin 325 mg once a day.

He has had minor past muscle pulls, the last episode occurring 2 years ago. He did not seek medical intervention but let "nature" take its course. He has never had pain this severe.

T A S K S

1. Based on the information you have, develop a list of differential diagnoses.

2. What information or symptoms in the history would make you consider (or not consider) the following as a cause of this patient's back pain?
A. Muscle pull or strain
B. Sciatica

C. Herniated disk
D. Vertebral dislocation
E. Abdominal aortic aneurysm
F. Degenerative joint disease of the spine
G. Renal calculi
H. Prostatitis
I. Pyelonephritis

3. On what components of the physical examination (PE) should you concentrate?

4. What findings on the PE would lead you to believe this injury is serious?

5. What special PE maneuvers are done to help in evaluating back pain?

PHYSICAL EXAMINATION

General: Well-developed, well-nourished African-American man in no apparent distress

Vital signs: Pulse 78, regular; Respirations 12, regular; Temperature 99.2°F (oral); Blood pressure 138/84; Weight 190 lb; Height 5′10″

Lungs: Clear to percussion and auscultation

Heart: Regular rate and rhythm; normal S1 and S2; no murmurs, rubs, or gallops

Abdomen: Mildly obese; active bowel sounds in all quadrants; nontender; no masses, organomegaly, or bruits

Genitalia: Circumcised penis; descended testicles; no hernias

Back: Normal spinal curvature; no costovertebral angle tenderness; tenderness in the paraspinal musculature of L2–L5 and over the sacroiliac joints; mild tenderness in the middle of the right buttock; musculoskeletal movements are as follows:

Back: Flexion to 20°, limited by tenderness; extension to 20°, limited by tenderness; right lateral bend to 80°; left lateral bend to 60°, limited by tenderness; rotation of shoulder, full without eliciting tenderness

Neck: Full range of motion (FROM); strength in all directions is 5/5

Hip: Full passive range of motion bilaterally; straight leg raise to 80° on the left; straight leg raise to 60° on right, limited by tenderness in the back; strength 5/5 in all directions, but extension causes discomfort in the back

Knees: FROM actively and passively; strength 5/5 for flexion and extension

Ankles: FROM actively and passively; strength 5/5 in all directions

Reflexes: 2+/4 and bilaterally equal at the patellar and Achilles' tendons; plantar reflex is down

Sensation: Intact soft touch, vibratory sense, and sharp/dull discrimination

Rectal: Prostate slightly enlarged, smooth, without mass/nodule, non-tender; guaiac test results negative

T A S K S

1. Based on this PE, modify your list of differential diagnoses.

2. Was a rectal examination necessary? Why or why not?

3. What findings in the history and PE would lead you to suspect any of the following conditions:
   A. Drug-seeking behavior
   B. Fracture of vertebra
   C. Ankylosing spondylitis
   D. Meningitis
   E. Herniated or ruptured disk
   F. Nonspinal cause of pain
   G. Degenerative joint disease of the spine
   H. Any of the conditions listed in the second set of tasks
   I. Prostate disease

4. What laboratory or other studies would you like to obtain?

5. Justify each of the tests you choose.

6. If you believe the diagnosis is low back pain secondary to sprain or strain, what is the appropriate treatment? Remember that treatment is more than medication. You should address activity, exercise, heat/cold, pain relief, return to work, prognosis, expectation of problem course, length of time to return to normal activities and full work status, medications and their side effects, and so forth.

7. Your patient would like to see the local chiropractor for manipulation. What do you tell him?

8. What are the criteria for referral to a back specialist?

9. Should his routine medications be changed?

10. What are the signs and symptoms that indicate more serious problems than muscle sprain or strain?

GENERAL DISCUSSION

Low back pain is one of the most common reasons that patients seek medical attention. It is a leading cause of disability and a major contributor to health-care costs. It is often overtreated, and its exact cause is frequently misdiagnosed. Effective treatment for most low back pain includes alterations in activity, low-stress exercise, pain relief, activity as tolerated, and time. Patient education is key because it takes 4 to 6 weeks for most back pain to resolve. Routine x-rays of the back (Fig. 10–1) generally show only age-related changes and are not necessary unless there is some indication of more severe problems. Patients who do not improve with conservative treatment should be evaluated further, and referral should be considered.

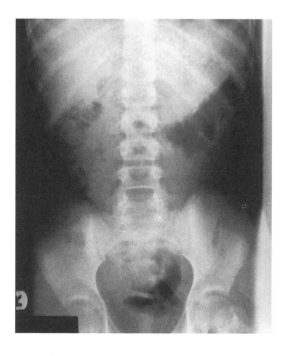

FIGURE 10–1 Anteroposterior (AP) x-ray of the lumbar spine showing age-related arthritic changes. Such images are not necessary for the diagnosis and treatment of most low back pain.

A key to evaluation is the recognition of serious conditions beyond the more common types of back strain and sprain. Some "red flags" for further evaluation include a history of direct trauma, signs or symptoms of infection, signs or symptoms of neoplasm, loss of sensation or function, worsening symptoms, changes in neurological functioning or examination, bowel or bladder dysfunction, and failure to improve.[1]

REFERENCE

1. Bigos SJ, et al. The new thinking on low-back pain. *Patient Care.* July 15, 1995.

SUGGESTED READING

Snider RK, ed. *Essentials of Musculoskeletal Care.* Rosemont, IL: American Academy of Orthopaedic Surgeons; 1997:490–546.

Resource Notes

List all the references you used for this case.

"I've Been Coughing a Lot."

BARBARA A. LYONS, MA, PA-C

BACKGROUND

You work in an urgent care clinic.

PATIENT HISTORY

The patient is Rose Anderson, a 62-year-old married white woman. She has a 3-day history of cough and fever. She lives with her husband in a house on the edge of Goliad, Texas. She is in your area visiting family over the New Year's holiday and presents to your clinic a few days after New Year's Day. About 3 days ago, she experienced the acute onset of cough with associated shortness of breath and fever with shaking chills. Her cough is productive, but she does not know its color because she has not looked at her sputum. The illness seemed to "knock her off her feet" and right into bed. She has not eaten well over the past few days, with soup and juice as her main food sources. She has been mildly anorectic but has not vomited or had diarrhea. She has taken extra-strength acetaminophen for her fever and an over-the-counter (OTC) cough suppressant for her cough, but neither is helping much. She also has taken a cough and cold preparation before going to bed to help her get some rest, but it hasn't helped much either.

T A S K S

1. With consideration of the foregoing presenting history, what additional history would you seek?

2. Even with this abbreviated history, what are some diagnoses you should begin to consider?

3. What factors should you consider relative to:
   A. The patient's age
   B. Her gender
   C. Her geographical risks (for example, where is her hometown of Goliad, Texas?)
   D. Her environmental or occupational exposures
   E. The diseases prevalent at this time of year

4. What are the effects, side effects, and interactions of the medications she is taking?

5. What causes shaking chills?

6. What causes people to cough?

7. How is cough controlled?

8. What is the significance of elevated temperature?

9. What is considered a fever?

10. What are the symptoms of the following, and how do they differ: upper respiratory infection (URI), common cold, influenza, bronchitis, and pneumonia?

ADDITIONAL HISTORY

Mrs. Anderson felt well and was enjoying her vacation with her son and his wife. Three nights ago, she awoke from sleep feeling warm, had one chill, and began to cough during the night. She slept intermittently the remainder of the night. Generally, she did not feel well on awakening, was warm, and had some joint aches. The cough continued. By the afternoon, her oral temperature was 102°F, and her cough increased in intensity and frequency. Acetaminophen lowered her fever. She thinks by that night her cough was productive. She was weak, having chills and paroxysms of coughing. She has taken the medications described with little relief. Her cough has worsened, and her temperature has not been below 101°F since yesterday. She is short of breath, especially during coughing spells. She has never had anything like this before.

The patient and her husband raise birds as the husband's retirement job. Mrs. Anderson smokes one pack of cigarettes per day and has since she was 18 years old. She does not drink alcohol except for an occasional glass of wine on holidays. She has never taken any illegal drugs and has never injected anything. She broke her wrist at age 25 when she fell from a horse. The injury healed without complications, and she had no sequelae from this incident. She is current with her immunizations, having been reimmunized with tetanus just before their "good" insurance was terminated upon her husband's retirement 2 years ago. She gets a yearly "flu shot" at the local pharmacy each autumn because it costs only five dollars. This year she received her shot in mid-October.

She has a history of grief reaction following the death of a son as an infant, for which she sought pastoral counseling. This occurred about 30 years ago, and although she is sometimes sad about it (generally around the anniversary of the infant's death), she feels she has dealt well with her grief. She eats well (three square meals per day), cooks low-fat meals, and uses plenty of vegetables from her garden. She is otherwise healthy, experienced menopause at age 51, and is taking hormone replacement therapy (HRT)—Premarin 0.625 mg per day—as well as a daily calcium supplement. She takes glucosamine for arthritis in her knees and is pleased with the results. She uses no other medications, herbals, or home remedies. She had a hysterectomy without complications at age 52 because of fibroids. She has had no blood transfusions. She is allergic to sulfa drugs, which make her break out in an itchy rash.

Mrs. Anderson has been a housewife all her married life. Though she has never been employed outside the home, she has helped out with the chores on their 5-acre farm. She is G3 P3 Ab0 LC2. She has a married 28-year-old daughter with two children. The daughter's family just concluded a visit to the patient's home over Christmas; during that time, one of the patient's grandchildren had a runny nose. Mrs. Anderson is now visiting her son, his wife, and child. She is in a mutually monogamous sexual relationship with her husband but declines to discuss her sex life any further, so as to maintain her privacy.

T A S K S

1. Based on the information you have, modify your list of potential diagnoses.

2. What are the patient's risk factors for respiratory system disease?

3. Does anything in her history raise your suspicion of some unusual respiratory disease?

4. What other organ system disease or dysfunction could account for her symptoms?

5. Could she have influenza despite having received an immunization for it this year?

6. What effects could her prescription and nonprescription medications have on her health or on this problem?

7. Does raising birds add to her respiratory risk for avian-related diseases?

8. What are the key points in her history?

9. Considering that all aspects of the physical examination (PE) are important, on what organ systems should you concentrate?

10. List each component of the PE, and describe what you would look for or examine.

11. What does the influenza vaccine protect against? (Be specific—what strains?) Should she have had the "pneumonia" vaccine? Should she be tested for tuberculosis (TB)?

PHYSICAL EXAMINATION

General: The patient sits on the examining table. She is obviously breathing fast and coughs frequently and deeply. She appears acutely ill and in moderate distress.

Vital signs: Pulse 104, standing pulse 110; Respirations 25; Temperature 102°F (oral); Blood pressure 128/88, right arm, sitting; Weight 110 lb; Height 5'3"

Skin: Poor turgor with slow return on pinch; no abnormal lesions

Head: Normocephalic; atraumatic

Eyes: Pupils equal, round, reactive to light and accommodation (PERRLA); extraocular movements intact (EOMI); cornea without opacities; sclera anicteric; conjunctiva clear; funduscopic examination reveals flat disks, mild arteriovenous (AV) nicking without exudates or hemorrhages

Ears: External ear intact; no pain on motion of pinna; external auditory canals (EACs) partially obstructed by cerumen; tympanic membrane (TM) visible, intact with normal landmarks, and cone of light bilaterally

Nose: Patent nares; moist and pinkish-red mucosa; no discharge from the turbinates

Mouth: No upper teeth (has dentures); bottom teeth intact and in good repair; pink and slightly dry mucosa with no lesions; cranial nerves IX and X intact

Throat: No lesions; no tonsillar enlargement

Chest:

> *Inspection:* No lesions; respiratory effort normal but tachypneic; no use of accessory muscles with respiration

> *Palpation:* No abnormalities palpated; no pain on palpation; fremitus increased over the right upper to middle fields

> *Percussion:* Dull to percussion over right upper to middle lobe; other areas resonant to percussion

> *Auscultation:* Vesicular breath sounds with rhonchi on forced expiration; fine, hard-to-hear rales at right base; loud rales in right middle field

Heart: Tachycardia (100) with regular rhythm; no murmurs, rubs, or gallops

Abdomen: Flat and nondistended with active bowel sounds; no hepatosplenomegaly or masses felt; no rebound

Neurologic: No obvious or gross central or peripheral deficits

Extremities: Yellowish stains on right fingers; no deformity of extremities; capillary refill less than 2 seconds; no splinter hemorrhages; no clubbing

Mental status: Oriented to person, place, time, and situation

T A S K S

1. List the pertinent findings (positive and negative) from the PE.

2. Based on the history and PE, redevelop your list of differential diagnoses for this patient.

3. What laboratory tests, diagnostic studies, imaging studies, and so forth do you want to order for this patient? As you consider these items, list what you will gain from each that will help you with diagnosis or management.

LABORATORY TESTS AND DIAGNOSTIC STUDIES

The patient may need other tests, but the following would form a basis for diagnosis and future monitoring:

1. Complete blood count (CBC) shows that white blood cells (WBCs) are 14,400/μL with a shift to the left.
2. Sputum gram stain shows numerous WBCs and gram-positive cocci that are too numerous to count. (Sputum would also be cultured and tested for sensitivity, but data would not be available for 3 to 5 days.)
3. Pulse oximeter shows that O_2 saturation is 94%, and pulse is 102.
4. Arterial blood gases (ABGs) are within normal limits.
5. Chest x-ray (Fig. 11–1) shows right upper lobe consolidation.

T A S K

Redefine your list of diagnoses based on all the information you have.

AUTHOR'S DIAGNOSIS

Your list should include community-acquired pneumonia, which is the primary diagnosis for this patient. Subsequent findings may change that diagnosis, but based on the presentation, this diagnosis is the most likely.

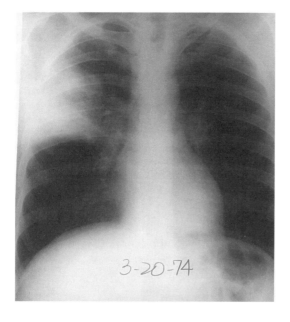

FIGURE 11–1 Chest x-ray.

T A S K S

1. What is the management of this problem?

2. Does this patient need to be hospitalized?

3. What types of pneumonia have the kind of findings shown on this chest x-ray?

4. What treatment would you suggest for this patient in her current condition?

5. What is the most cost-efficient, effective treatment?

6. How would the treatment of the patient differ if she were hospitalized versus treated as an outpatient?

7. How do the costs compare?

8. How would you determine which treatment would be most effective?

9. What would be the patient's prognosis if she were hospitalized versus treated as an outpatient?

10. What factors should you consider if her treatment course and progress do not proceed as expected?

GENERAL DISCUSSION

Community-acquired pneumonia affects 1% of the general population in the United States annually. It accounts for major health-care costs and is still one of the most common causes of death.[1] *Streptococcus pneumoniae* is the most common causative organism, but the epidemiology of pneumonia is changing, and providers need to be aware of all the organisms that can cause pneumonia. Approaches to the assessment and management of patients suspected of having pneumonia differ. History is important, and the assessment of risk factors and cofactors must be considered. The chest x-ray is still considered the gold standard for diagnosis. Sputum culture and sensitivity identify the causative agent. Controversy over treatment is widespread, and you need to refer to recent literature for the current recommendations. Risk factors for pulmonary disease, including HIV risk, should be investigated.

REFERENCE

1. Cross JT. Bacterial pneumonia. In Rakel RE, ed. *Conn's Current Therapy.* Philadelphia: WB Saunders; 2000:209–213.

Resource Notes

List all the references you used for this case.

"I Think My Husband Has Alzheimer's."

RICHARD R. RAHR, EdD, PA-C • VIRGINIA A. RAHR, EdD, ANP

BACKGROUND

You work in a family practice clinic near an academic health science center.

PATIENT HISTORY

John Smithers is a 63-year-old white man who worked at the academic health science center for 33 years until his retirement 1 year ago. At age 22, John started at the medical school as an orderly, transporting patients in the x-ray department. In 1967, he attended the certificate program at the teaching hospital for 2 years to become an x-ray technologist. He passed his American Registry of Radiologic Technology (ARRT) Board Examinations in 1969 and was hired as a staff x-ray technologist at the center hospital. John advanced to his department's top position, that of chief technologist, which he held for 17 years. By the time he retired, he supervised 60 employees. Through his retirement plan, John now receives 70% of his former salary. He always wanted to retire so he could play golf and tennis each day with close friends. In addition, John has always wanted to travel to Europe, South America, and Hawaii.

John married his wife, Joan, 10 years ago. They have no children. Joan was a student technologist when they met, and their wedding took place following her graduation from the radiologic technology program at the medical school. Joan, who is 25 years younger than John, is chief technologist in a private practice radiology office. She loves her job and the income it yields.

Since his retirement, John has wanted her to quit and travel with him. This issue has caused friction between them because of the pressure that John has placed on Joan.

Joan has brought John to see you (both are your patients and have been relatively healthy) about John's recent behavior. She states, "I think my husband has Alzheimer's." She provides most of the following history. When he retired, John played golf and tennis each day for 3 months with his retired friends. Then he began staying home and sleeping until noon. Now when Joan comes home from work at 5 PM, John is still in his pajamas. He stays up late at night watching television because he has problems falling asleep. John told Joan that he lost $100,000 recently in the stock market because of some bad investments. He has gained 60 pounds during the last 6 months, largely because he eats all day, has stopped playing tennis, and is not doing any physical activities. He bathes infrequently, sometimes less than once a week. He has trouble remembering what day it is and balancing his checkbook. He has had no desire for sexual relations for the past 3 months; his activity, thinking, speech, and memory also have slowed during this same period. Joan has noticed that John has been turning up the thermostat at home, and he often says he is very cold. He keeps a blanket over himself all day. He has complained of chronic constipation and is taking a fiber compound twice each day for relief.

John says very little, and you ask Joan to leave the room while you talk to him. The first comment he makes is that he believes Joan is having an affair at work with one of the radiologists. He believes that she will ask him for a divorce, and if she does, John does not know what he will do.

T A S K S

1. What additional history do you need from John?

2. What are your tentative differential diagnoses?

3. Is there a need to make a quick diagnosis for this patient?

4. Do you need a family history from John?

5. Is a medication history important?

6. What additional review of systems (ROS) do you need?

7. Would a psychiatric history be helpful?

8. What are the signs and symptoms of Alzheimer's disease?

ADDITIONAL HISTORY

While making the bed last night after coming home from work, Joan found the family gun, loaded, under John's pillow. She angrily quizzed John about the loaded gun under his pillow. John began to cry uncontrollably, saying he just felt worthless and was thinking of killing himself. He showed her a half-written suicide note that contained all his suspicions about Joan preparing to leave him for her coworker. John stated that he would kill himself if Joan left. Joan made it very clear to John that she was not having an affair at work nor was she thinking of leaving him. They agreed to see someone in your office in the morning. Joan lay awake all night watching John, so he would not do anything to hurt himself. She had hidden the gun and the car keys.

During John's outburst, he told Joan that he feared he was becoming like his mother, who had multiple fits of depression and suicide attempts before being placed on medication. John's mother was admitted many times to the psychiatric hospital while he was in high school. His mother's depressive episodes were so bad that she would go for days without speaking to anyone or leaving her room. After she was placed on medication, she improved markedly. She died, however, in a motor vehicle collision under suspicious circumstances. Her death was ruled as accidental. John was also concerned with "losing his mind" as his father had in his eighties.

John has received pharmacological treatment for hypertension, which usually controls his blood pressure well. He is currently taking hydrochlorothiazide/triamterene, 25/37.5 mg twice a day; enalapril, 10 mg once a day; and propranolol, 40 mg three times a day. His medication regimen has not changed for the last 5 years. John has been complaining about dry skin, thickening of his hair, and constipation. In the last few days, his appetite has decreased, which is a change from his period of overeating. John has been getting up four to five times each night to urinate.

T A S K S

1. Would you like to ask any additional historical questions?

2. How would you refine your list of differential diagnoses?

3. What are the drug interactions for the medications John is taking?

4. What are the contraindications and adverse effects of the drugs he is taking?

5. What are the important components of the physical examination (PE)?

6. What are the components of the mental and physical examination for altered mental status?

PHYSICAL EXAMINATION

General: This 63-year-old white man is in no acute distress.

Vital signs: Pulse 92; Respirations 16; Temperature 99°F (oral); Blood pressure 160/88; Weight 240 lb; Height 5'10"

Skin: No lesions, ecchymosis, pallor, or rubor

HEENT: Normocephalic; atraumatic; pupils equal, round, reactive to light and accommodation (PERRLA); conjunctiva clear; sclera white; extraocular movements intact (EOMI); funduscopic examination shows grade one Keith Wagner changes with arterial narrowing and arteriovenous (AV) nicking, sharp disk margins, no papilledema; patent external auditory canal; tympanic membranes (TMs) have tympanosclerosis bilaterally, normal cone of light, normal position and color; nasal mucosa pink and moist; septum without deviation; pink and moist mouth; oral pharynx without lesions, swelling, or exudate; pink and moist buccal mucosa and gums; teeth in good repair but need cleaning; foul breath

Neck: Normal carotid pulses without bruits; normal thyroid without masses; trachea midline; no nodes, no jugular venous distention (JVD); no masses; full range of motion (FROM) to the neck; muscle strength 5/5 to extension, flexion, lateral movement, and rotation

Chest: Clear to auscultation and percussion

Heart: Normal S1 and S2 with no evidence of gallops or murmurs

Abdomen: Active bowel sounds; no organomegaly, bruits, or masses; no palpable kidneys or tenderness

Extremities: Peripheral pulses (dorsalis pedis [DP], posterior tibia [PT], femoral, radial, brachial) 2+/4 and bilaterally equal; no edema or swelling; normal turgor, temperature, and texture of skin; FROM of upper and lower extremities

Rectal/genitourinary: Asymmetrical testicles; patent meatus; no evidence of hernia; normal anal sphincter tone; no hemorrhoids; guaiac-negative stool

Lymph: No evidence of edema or swelling

Neurologic: Patient oriented to time, place, and person; Romberg test results negative; normal gait and cerebellar functions; reflexes 2+ and bilaterally equal; cranial nerves II–XII intact; muscular strength 5/5 and bilaterally equal; smell and taste not tested; pin prick, hot/cold, and vibratory testing within normal limits

Mini-Mental Status Examination score: 28

Geriatric Depression Scale score: 10

T A S K S

1. Do you need to perform any other components of the PE?

2. What are the Mini-Mental Status Examination and Geriatric Depression Scale? What do the results mean?

3. Does the patient need a full mental status examination? If yes, describe the examination.

4. Refine your differential diagnoses list. Prioritize the list by problem.

5. What laboratory tests or diagnostic studies would you like to obtain?

6. Would any special tests help you arrive at a solution?

LABORATORY TESTS AND DIAGNOSTIC STUDIES

1. Complete blood count (CBC) is within normal limits.
2. Urinalysis (UA) is normal except for trace protein.
3. Chest x-ray is normal except for mild osteoarthritic changes of the spine.
4. Electrocardiogram (EKG) is within normal limits.

T A S K S

1. Does this patient require a computed tomography (CT) scan of the head?

2. Does this patient require thyroid function tests?

3. Do you need to order a serum protein electrophoresis test?

4. Do you need to order a drug screening for this patient?

5. What would you learn from each of the above?

COMMON DIFFERENTIALS TO ENTERTAIN

- Depression with suicide ideation
- Hypothyroidism
- Brain tumor
- Medication side effect
- Marital discord
- Hypertension
- Osteoarthritis
- Obesity
- Benign prostatic hypertrophy (BPH)

T A S K S

Assume a primary diagnosis of depression for this patient. Based on this diagnosis, consider the following:

1. Should John be hospitalized?

2. Should he be referred to a psychiatrist immediately?

3. Should you attempt to counsel him on an ongoing basis?

4. Should you prescribe antidepressants immediately?

5. Should you consult your supervising physician?

GENERAL DISCUSSION

Depression, a primary mood disorder, manifests itself by depressed mood, decreased interest and pleasure in formerly enjoyed activities, poor appetite, sleep disorders, fatigue, poor memory, suicide ideation, weight loss or gain, poor concentration, lack of interest in hobbies or habits, and poor self-image. It occurs in 5% to 20% of all persons at some time in their lives. Depression is thought to be related to a decrease in the dopamine, serotonin, and norepinephrine receptor-neurotransmitter function. It tends to develop in patients who have a positive family history of depression.

The rate of depression is greater in women than in men. There are many risk factors for increased incidence of depression. Patients with increased stress, insomnia, recent myocardial infarction (MI), back pain, or migraine cephalgia will have increased bouts of depression. Depression is prevalent in older adults, recently retired individuals, and patients with back pain, chronic pain, or chronic illnesses.

The signs and symptoms of depression can mimic many diseases, and many diseases may cause or have depression as a component of their presentations. Depression commonly is associated with hypothyroidism or hyperthyroidism. It is also very common in patients with substance abuse disorders. The withdrawal of cocaine, alcohol, or marijuana can trigger an episode of depression. Depression is a common side effect of everyday, frequently used prescription drugs, such as antihypertensives, hormones, sedatives, antihistamines, anticonvulsants, antiparkinsonian drugs, cardiac medications, anti-infectives, antineoplastics, and nonsteroidal anti-inflammatory drugs (NSAIDs).[1] Patients with chronic fatigue syndrome also have a very high incidence of depression. Long-standing chronic renal or liver failure may lead to depression, as may diabetes mellitus (DM).

The assessment of patients with depression will require the use of some type of medical assessment scale (for example, Beck's Depression Scale, Children's Depression Index [CDI], and Criteria for Epidemologic Studies [CES] Depression Scale) to quantify in points the likelihood or severity of a diagnosis of depression. Relatively new drugs that can be used to treat depression include Zoloft, Paxil, Wellbutrin, Effexor, and Prozac. Pharmacologic treatment for depression will require 6 months to 2 years of constant ingestion for the desired effect. Patients will not experience the therapeutic effect until at least 2 to 3 weeks after they begin taking such medications.

The major factor to watch for in all patients with depression is suicide ideation that leads to a suicide plan. All patients with serious suicide ideation need close evaluation. All patients with a suicide plan require admittance to a locked unit with close psychiatric observation. Medication for depression may, after 2 to 3 weeks, give the depressed patient enough energy to commit suicide.

Providers should immediately refer any patients with serious suicide ideation or a suicide plan to a psychiatrist. They should discuss this with the patient, the family, and their supervising physicians. Those who are licensed to do so and have the skill and experience necessary should counsel for depression.

T A S K S

1. State all the risk factors for depression.

2. List all the signs and symptoms for depression.

3. Pick a depression scale (such as Beck's Depression Scale) to use when screening your patients.

4. Learn how to carefully ask each patient about suicide ideation or suicide plans.

5. Know the immediate steps that you need to take when a patient has suicide plans.

6. Learn how to educate patients who have frequent bouts of depression about the common signs and symptoms that need treatment.

7. Research the newest drugs used to treat acute and chronic depression.

REFERENCE

1. Edmunds MW, Mayhew MS. *Pharmacology for the Primary Care Provider.* St. Louis: Mosby; 2000:604.

SUGGESTED READING

Mannshreck, DD. Depression. In Dambro MR, ed. *Griffith's 5-Minute Clinical Consult 2000.* Philadelphia: Lippincott Williams & Wilkins; 2000:294–295.

Resource Notes

List all the references you used for this case.

"I Was Coughing and Wheezing Last Night."

KAREN S. STEPHENSON, MS, PA-C

BACKGROUND

You work in a family practice clinic in a medium-sized city.

PATIENT HISTORY

Tiffany Morgan, a 10-year-old African-American girl, comes to the clinic with her aunt and father because of the onset of nocturnal coughing and wheezing. Tiffany states emphatically, "I was coughing and wheezing last night." She also has a 2-week history of nasal congestion, rhinorrhea, and sore throat. She and her father deny any episodes of fever.

T A S K S

1. What additional historical questions would you ask, especially in the review of systems (ROS)?

2. What are the common causes of coughing in Tiffany's age group?

3. What is the usual history for a child with asthma?

4. What are the risks factors for developing asthma?

5. What are some common evaluation and treatment approaches for asthma?

ADDITIONAL HISTORY

Tiffany's usual cough is normally nonproductive, although she does produce yellow-green mucus upon retiring and just as she gets up each morning. Her aunt has noticed halitosis and possible hearing loss. Tiffany does not complain of nasal itching, but her father and aunt have observed her rubbing her nose frequently. Her family is unaware of possible causes but notice that symptoms worsen with cold or damp weather. They also have noticed that Tiffany sometimes coughs after running or riding her bicycle. The father smokes but not in the house. Tiffany takes no medications regularly, although her aunt has given her several over-the-counter (OTC) cough preparations recently, usually at night. Her aunt does not give Tiffany such medicine before school because they cause drowsiness. These OTC medications have not relieved her symptoms, even for the first few hours after she has taken them.

This is the first time you are seeing Tiffany, but she has come to the clinic and the emergency room (ER) for similar problems in the past. Her dad reports that he had similar problems as a child, including allergies and asthma. There is no known history of heart disease, congenital defects, cystic fibrosis, immunodeficiency, or recurrent bronchitis. Tiffany denies swallowing any foreign body.

Tiffany was born at a large hospital in another city. Her parents were divorced before she was born. Her father knows little of her early childhood because Tiffany lived with her mother in a large city about 1 hour away for the first 3 years of her life. Her family denies any knowledge of medical problems, surgeries, injuries, broken bones, or allergies. Her aunt and dad are unaware of any problems with the mother's pregnancy or childbirth and believe that Tiffany's development has been normal. Tiffany is current on her immunizations.

Tiffany is in the fourth grade and states she had As and Bs on her last report card. She lives with her dad and visits her relatives often. She has no further contact with her mother. She says she likes school and spending recess with her friends because she is an only child. She seems well-adjusted for her age and happy with her living arrangements. She enjoys playing with her cat.

T A S K S

1. Based on the historical information you have, develop a list of differential diagnoses.

2. What physical examination (PE) is necessary to confirm and rule out the differential diagnoses that you are considering?

3. What is the PE specifically for the upper and lower respiratory tracts?

4. What are the indicators of upper and lower airway disease on PE?

5. What considerations should you give to her family/domestic situation?

PHYSICAL EXAMINATION

General: The patient sits with her dad. She appears ill but answers questions readily.

Vital signs: Pulse 124; Respirations 24 (17 to 21 normal for her age); Temperature 99.6°F (oral); Blood pressure 100/60; Weight 75 lb; Height 57"

Skin: Warm and dry to the touch

Head: Normocephalic

Eyes: Pupils equal, round, reactive to light and accommodation (PERRLA); sclera anicteric; conjunctiva clear

Ears: External auditory canals (EACs) patent with some cerumen in the canal; tympanic membrane (TM) visible, gray, with light reflex; some injection in both TMs but no bulging or erythema noted; some decreased mobility to insufflation in both TMs

Nose: Patent nares; moist and pale mucosa; yellow-green discharge in each nostril; pain elicited upon percussion over both maxillary sinuses

Mouth: Teeth present and without obvious cavities; halitosis noted upon examination

Throat: No lesions; no tonsillar enlargement; no erythema or exudate

Chest:

> *Inspection:* No lesions; respiratory effort normal but tachypneic; no use of accessory muscles with respiration
>
> *Palpation:* No abnormalities or pain on palpation
>
> *Auscultation:* Expiratory wheezing heard over both lung fields; a few rhonchi heard but no rales; deep breathing precipitated coughing, which then cleared the rhonchi

Heart: Tachycardic with regular rhythm; no murmurs, rubs, or gallops

Abdomen: Flat, nondistended; bowel sounds active; no hepatosplenomegaly or masses felt; no rebound

Neurologic: No obvious or gross central or peripheral deficits

Extremities: No cyanosis or edema noted; capillary refill less than 2 seconds

Mental status: Oriented to person, place, time, and situation

T A S K S

1. Based on the additional information from the PE, refine your list of differential diagnoses.

2. What laboratory tests and diagnostic studies would you like to order?

3. For each test or special study you listed in task 2, describe what the results will confirm or negate in your differential. Ask yourself if the tests are absolutely necessary.

4. What is the cost of each test you ordered, and how long before the results are available?

LABORATORY TESTS AND DIAGNOSTIC STUDIES

1. Peak expiratory flow rate is 245.6 L/min.
2. Pulse oximetry reading is 95%.
3. The chest x-ray (Fig. 13–1A) shows increased perihilar markings and right middle lobe infiltrate, which cleared after treatment for asthma (Fig. 13–1B). Other common x-ray findings are shown in Figure 13–2.

T A S K S

1. How is a peak flow done? What is normal for Tiffany? How do patients use peak flow at home to monitor asthma?

2. What is pulse oximetry, and what can it tell you? Why should you check the patient's pulse when you evaluate the pulse oximetry reading?

3. What are the signs of asthma that can be seen on a chest x-ray? Are there any distinctive criteria for asthma?

4. What conflicts exist in the literature concerning the diagnosis of sinusitis by x-ray for adults and children? When do the sinuses develop, and when does clinical disease develop for each set of sinuses? How would you resolve these conflicts?

5. Which of the preceding tests are absolutely indicated for the evaluation of this child? Are there any additional tests that you might wish to obtain? State your rationale for these additional tests.

6. What are your differential diagnoses based on the history, PE, and laboratory and diagnostic information?

7. How has the addition of the diagnostic information helped to further narrow your diagnoses?

8. How will you treat Tiffany? (Remember medication, palliative treatment, patient education, follow-up, and the need to return.)

9. How will you monitor her disease?

10. What lifestyle changes will she and her family have to make?

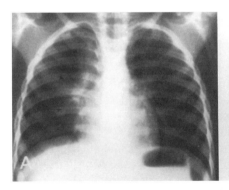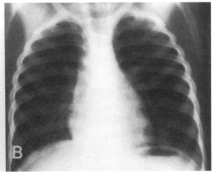

FIGURE 13–1 (*A*) An x-ray showing an infiltrate in the right middle lobe of a child with asthma. (*B*) The infiltrate disappears within 24 hours after the onset of treatment for asthma. This change is consistent with atelectasis rather than pneumonia. Although not everyone with asthma needs a second x-ray, the two views demonstrate the need to clarify whether a child with asthma has pneumonia or segmental atelectasis from bronchospasm. (From Swischuk LE. *Emergency Imaging of the Acutely Ill or Injured Child.* 4th ed. Philadelphia: Lippincott, Williams & Wilkins; 2000, pp. 82–88; reprinted with permission.)

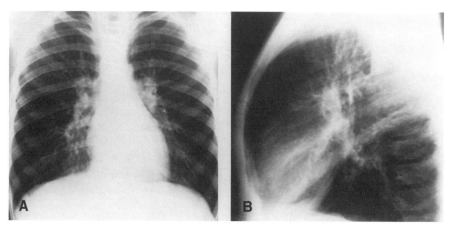

FIGURE 13-2 This x-ray demonstrates overaeration and perihilar/peribronchial markings, which are common radiographic findings for someone with asthma. (From Swischuk LE. *Emergency Imaging of the Acutely Ill or Injured Child.* 4th ed. Philadelphia: Lippincott, Williams & Wilkins; 2000, pp. 82–88; reprinted with permission.)

DIFFERENTIAL DIAGNOSES FOR WHEEZING

For older children, consider asthma; viral upper respiratory infection (URI); foreign body; gastroesophageal reflux; sinusitis (properly described as rhinosinusitis); atopy, including allergic rhinitis; immunodeficiency (IgG); and allergic bronchopulmonary aspergillosis.[1]

If your patient is an infant, then consider bronchopulmonary dysplasia (BPD), cystic fibrosis, tracheal obstruction, foreign body, gastroesophageal reflux, bronchiolitis, large airway obstruction, congenital or acquired cardiac disease, and congestive heart failure.[1,2]

If the patient is an adolescent, then consider asthma, allergic rhinitis, sinusitis, and allergic bronchopulmonary aspergillosis. A patient of any age can aspirate a foreign body or exhibit pulmonary edema.[1] Adolescents may smoke, which may precipitate wheezing in those with asthma. As the number of teens contracting human immunodeficiency virus (HIV) continues to increase, also consider *Pneumocystis carinii* pneumonia (PCP) as the cause of wheezing and shortness of breath (SOB) in sexually active teens.

T A S K S

1. What else should you consider about the diagnoses you believe are appropriate for this child?

2. What are the anatomical and physiological changes that occur in asthma?

3. Make a list of the categories of medications that can be used to treat asthma.

4. Review and discuss the lifestyle changes that families and individuals with asthma should make.

5. Find at least one recent flow sheet or algorithm for the evaluation, treatment, and management of asthma.

GENERAL DISCUSSION

After consideration of the history, PE, and laboratory and diagnostic studies, the most likely diagnosis for this child is exacerbation of asthma by allergic rhinitis and maxillary rhinosinusitis. Wheezing is a very common symptom in both children and adults. Although asthma commonly causes wheezing, other etiologies should not be automatically dismissed without due consideration for less likely causes. As noted under "Differential Diagnoses for Wheezing," the child's age should help guide the diagnoses under consideration.[1]

Tiffany has the classic symptoms for asthma: coughing and wheezing, especially at night, and noted with exercise or some other trigger. You should also seek a family history that is positive for atopy and be prepared for patients who describe recurrent bronchitis or pneumonia, especially with a family history of allergies or atopic dermatitis. (Patients may describe atopic dermatitis as "extremely dry skin" and call allergies "hay fever.") Some family members may not come forth with that history until the provider is explaining the treatment for the child. This patient has a mild exacerbation of her asthma; her pulse oximetry is above 92%, and her peak expiratory flow rate (PEFR) is at 80% of the predicted best based on her height in inches. Remember to check the patient's pulse when evaluating the pulse oximetric reading to confirm its accuracy.[3] Her initial chest x-ray (see Fig. 13–1A) reveals perihilar markings and an apparent consolidation that clears with treatment of asthma.

Tiffany also has a positive family history for IgE-mediated disease, and allergic rhinitis and rhinosinusitis are noted during today's visit. She has been treated for similar illnesses during previous ER visits. Chronic cough alone may be the only symptom for asthma, rather than cough and wheezing concurrently.[4] This condition, known as cough-variant asthma, is found in both children and adults.

This patient has no evidence of cardiac disease or any of the several conditions in infants that cause wheezing and would have been symptomatic earlier (that is, cystic fibrosis, BPD, bronchiolitis). She is unlikely to have unknowingly swallowed a foreign body, but that must be considered if the wheezing does not respond to therapy.

Tiffany's nasal mucosa is pale, as would be expected with allergic rhinitis. (It can also be violet.) Her aunt has seen her scratching and rubbing her nose, and her aunt and father have noticed for the past 2 weeks that whenever trigger factors such as weather changes have caused Tiffany to have rhinorrhea, it has been yellow-green. Other trigger factors to inquire about include exposure to pollens, grasses, dust mites, cockroaches, pollution, ozone, perfumes, and cigarette smoke. The presence of allergic rhinitis and yellow-green mucus in the nares for 2 weeks supports the diagnosis of rhinosinusitis. The duration of the discharge is more important than its color or characteristics.[4] URIs also may have purulent discharge, but in a URI the infection begins with clear, mucoid discharge, which becomes purulent and then returns to clear and mucoid over 7 to 10 days.

The purulent discharge indicates infection, but it alone does not differentiate between viral or bacterial causes. In one retrospective chart review that compared sinusitis with URI symptoms, several factors were identified as predictive of sinusitis: Sinus tenderness, sinus pressure, postnasal drainage, and discolored discharge explained 60% of the differences in diagnosis.[5] Other factors also found to be statistically significant included cough, maxillary toothache, headache, and abnormal transillumination. All were significant at the $p < .001$ level. Factors identified as indicating URI included nasal congestion, earache, fatigue, nausea, poor response to decongestants, and abnormal ear and lung examinations. (Most of the patients in this study were probably adults, although some must have been younger; the mean age for the URI group was 22 years, and one pediatric reference was cited.)

Even though the findings from this study may not apply directly to children, the study does support targeting those factors that can definitively separate two conditions that share symptoms. As the authors state: "This use of unreliable criteria may lead to misdiagnosis and inappropriate prescriptions for antibiotics."[5] The color of the rhinorrhea should not be used *alone* as the deciding factor for the use of antibiotics. Increasing resistance of *Streptococcus pneumoniae* to aminopenicillins and the increasing numbers of *Haemophilus influenzae* and *Moraxella (Branhamella) ca-*

tarrhalis that can produce beta-lactamase are the result of overuse of antibiotics, especially for URIs. These developments complicate the selection of antibiotics when needed for a bacterial infection, such as otitis or rhinosinusitis.

Treatment of asthma, allergic rhinitis, and maxillary rhinosinusitis is very intertwined. Allergic rhinitis, URIs, and maxillary rhinosinusitis can precipitate an asthmatic episode, and treatment of asthma must address the trigger factors to alleviate the patient's symptoms. Asthma is caused by an inflammatory response in the bronchial tree that is mediated by white blood cells. The inflammatory component must be addressed to bring asthma under control. Bronchodilators treat bronchospasm only after it has occurred. Steroids, sodium cromolyn, and leukotrienes, on the other hand, interfere with the bronchospasm from the time the antigen is first identified, so they can prevent or abort exacerbations of asthma. Daily PEFR monitoring and close monitoring of symptoms, especially coughing at night, can follow the status and treatment of asthma.[2] It is especially important that patients and parents understand that coughing may be the only sign or an early sign of worsening bronchospasm.

The PEFR and pulse oximetry indicate that Tiffany is experiencing an exacerbation of her asthma that best fits the definition of intermittent asthma.[6] She should initially be given nebulized treatments with albuterol every 20 to 30 minutes during the first hour. The vital signs, pulse oximetry, and PEFR should be followed closely during this period. If she is not improved, her treatment should become more intensive, with initiation of inhaled or systemic steroids. If her pulse oximetry stays at 93% or greater and her PEFR is at least 80% of the expected rate for her height, she can be maintained at this level. If not, her treatment should become more intensive. For a detailed description of the treatment of asthma, see the Web site sponsored by the National Institutes of Health.[6] A slightly different, more limited stepwise approach has also been outlined.[7]

The chest x-ray also assists in the diagnosis of asthma, but more important, it rules out complications of asthma and/or other conditions that may mimic asthma. Viral infections in the lower respiratory tract are the most common cause of an asthmatic exacerbation, whereas parenchymal consolidations, such as bacterial pneumonia, are not.[8] Viral infections in children with asthma may lead to segmental atelectasis, which may incorrectly be diagnosed as bacterial pneumonia. Treatment of the asthma leads to resolution of the atelectasis in as little as 24 hours. Pneumonia can be misdiagnosed in someone with asthma, especially if the patient is not wheezing at the time of exam. Overaeration and perihilar/peribronchial markings are also common findings during an asthmatic exacerbation (see Fig. 13–2). Chest x-rays are often done, looking for complications such as pneumonia or pneumothorax, but most films demonstrate the findings commonly noted with asthma. The ultimate decision to perform the chest x-ray, though, is left to the health-care professional and depends on the patient's response to the treatment intervention.

In addition, allergic rhinitis, sinusitis, and gastroesophageal reflux must also be brought under control. Topical nasosteroids and topical sodium cromolyn are effective at reducing allergic nasal symptoms.[9] Some young children are put off by the spraying action of the medications and may require systemic medications instead. Nonsedating antihistamines are preferred; even if first generation antihistamines are given at night, sedation can linger.[9] The same medications for allergic rhinitis can help to reduce inflammation at the os of the maxillary sinuses, preventing the development of rhinosinusitis. For patients who continue to have nocturnal symptoms (especially cough), gastroesophageal reflux may be a contributing factor and should be treated. By addressing both the symptoms of asthma and the concurrent conditions that may precipitate it, patients can remain symptom free, anticipate exacerbations of asthma, and maintain their daily activities.

REFERENCES

1. Torda W. Asthma. In Dershewitz RA, ed. *Ambulatory Pediatric Care.* 3rd ed. Philadelphia: Lippincott-Raven; 1999:329–335.
2. Dorkin HL. Bronchiolitis. In Dershewitz RA, ed. *Ambulatory Pediatric Care,* 3rd ed. Philadelphia: Lippincott-Raven; 1999:847–850.
3. Siberry GK, Iannone R. *The Harriet Lane Handbook.* 15th ed. St. Louis: Mosby-Year Book, Inc; 2000:535.
4. Wald ER. Chronic sinusitis in children. *J Pediatr.* 1995;127:339–347.
5. Hueston WJ, Eberlein C, Johnson D, Mainous AG. Criteria used by clinicians to differentiate sinusitis from viral upper respiratory tract infection. *J Fam Pract.* 1998;46:487–492.
6. National Asthma Education and Prevention Program Expert Panel Report 2: Guidelines for the Diagnosis and Management of Asthma. Bethesda, MD: National Heart, Lung, and Blood Institute; 1997. NIH Publication No. 97–4051. Available at: http://www.nhlbi.nih.gov/guidelines/asthma/asthgdln.pdf
7. Busse WW. A 47-year-old woman with severe asthma. *JAMA.* 2000;284:2225–2233.
8. Swischuk LE. *Emergency Imaging of the Acutely Ill or Injured Child.* 4th ed. Philadelphia: Lippincott, Williams & Wilkins; 2000:82–88.
9. International Rhinitis Management Working Group. International Consensus Report on the diagnosis and management of rhinitis. *Allergy.* 1994;49(19 Suppl):1–34.

Resource Notes

List all the references you used for this case.

"One from a Wreck!"

FRANCES COULSON, MS, PA-C

Author's Note: This case has a different presentation than other cases in the book. Although much emergency care occurs simultaneously, practice progresses in a linear fashion. To work through this case, you will need some background knowledge of emergency care. We suggest you review basic life support (BLS), advanced cardiac life support (ACLS), and advanced trauma life support (ATLS), or at a minimum, find and study an emergency medicine algorithm or flow sheet.

BACKGROUND

You are part of the medical staff—one physician (MD) and one physician assistant (PA) on a 12-hour shift—of a small 60-bed hospital.

PATIENT HISTORY

While you are working in the emergency department (ED), a pickup truck pulls into the ambulance entrance. Two men announce that they have the victim of a motor vehicle collision in the back of their truck. Your supervising physician just left to attend to a patient with cardiac arrest. He will be unavailable for consult or help until the code is completed.

T A S K

What do you do first?

The initial evaluation of the patient before moving him should include a brief visual survey to determine a rough estimate of age, size, sex, color, and alertness. Approaching the patient, you should perform this survey as a brief, almost unconscious evaluation. The initial action is to check airway, breathing, and circulation (remember the ABCs) and level of consciousness. Intervention is to open and secure the airway and to make sure the patient is breathing and the heart is beating.

T A S K

Review the interventions necessary if the patient is in full cardiac arrest.

From this brief examination, you find that the patient is a white male who appears to be in his fifties. He is approximately 5′8″ and about 220 lb. He is pale, cold to the touch, and moaning unintelligibly. His respirations are 26 breaths per minute, and his radial pulse is weakly palpable at 130 beats per minute. Additionally, you note dried and fresh blood on his face and on the left upper pant leg.

T A S K

What should you do now based on the preceding initial evaluation?

At this point, your interventions should focus on correcting anything life threatening, such as opening the airway, stopping any obvious severe bleeding, covering a sucking chest wound, and decompressing a tension pneumothorax. These basic interventions serve as necessities to prevent the patient's immediate death.

T A S K S

1. Should you take any specific actions as other medical personnel and equipment arrive?

2. Dilemma: Should you perform further evaluation before moving the patient, or should you move the patient to the trauma room, which has adequate lighting and readily available equipment?

3. How should a trauma victim be secured prior to movement?

A backboard, cervical (C) collar, and a bed have been brought out to move the patient inside.

T A S K S

1. What is the proper way to move this patient onto the bed?

2. Upon moving the patient into the trauma room, what is the next appropriate action by all involved? Review the primary survey, and describe what you are looking for and how to manage the problems you find.

3. What are the team members responsible for doing during this time?

4. What information should you gather from the men who brought the patient to the ED?

5. Develop a list of questions you should ask.

The two men who brought the patient to the ED give information. They found the patient's automobile with its front end slammed into a tree on an icy curve about 10 miles outside of town. When they opened the door of the patient's car, some empty beer cans fell out; the patient was not wearing his seat belt. They pulled the patient from the driver's side and placed him in the bed of their pickup. The patient was mumbling, but they could not understand what he was saying. They noticed that the windshield was broken in a circular fashion and that the steering wheel was bent. There was no air bag. They saw no other victims. They did not witness the actual accident, so they do not know how long the patient had been sitting there before they arrived. They do not remember seeing steam escaping from the hood area, nor did they feel the hood to see if it was still warm.

T A S K S

1. Develop a list of potential injuries and medical conditions the patient may have as a result of the information you have.

2. What do you do now?

Many things need to be done. All members of the team should already know their duties and be working on them. These duties include drawing blood for laboratory studies and establishing large-bore intravenous (IV) catheters with Ringer's lactate solution or normal saline (NS), typing and crossmatching, and so forth. The patient's clothes should be removed by cutting them off to reveal any hidden injuries. The patient's extremities should be restrained. The bed should be placed in the Trendelenburg position if the patient's pulse is weak or absent. Electrocardiogram (EKG) leads should be applied. The team leader or respiratory therapist, if present, should take control of the airway, and the team leader should do a proper primary survey and secondary survey.

T A S K S

1. What is a "primary" survey?

2. What is a "secondary" survey?

3. How big is a large-bore IV catheter?

4. How fast should the IVs initially be allowed to flow?

PRIMARY SURVEY

During the primary survey, you find a laceration to the patient's head at the hairline with active bleeding. You find that the patient opens his eyes to verbal commands, responds with inappropriate words, and pushes your hand away from painful areas. His airway is intact, and breathing continues at 26 breaths per minute. A non-rebreather mask has been placed on the patient with O_2 at 12 L/min. The medical technician is cutting off the patient's clothing. The patient's neck veins are not full, and his trachea is midline. You notice splinting, bruising, and pain with palpation over the lower left chest wall around the anterior axillary line. There is an arc-shaped contusion to the left anterior chest. There are no open wounds or blood on the chest. Lung sounds are diminished over the painful area but clear elsewhere.

T A S K S

1. With this information, is any intervention needed immediately before moving to the rest of the primary survey?

2. What is the patient's Glasgow Coma Scale score (Table 14–1)? What does the Glasgow Coma score mean?

TABLE 14–1   GLASGOW COMA SCALE

Examination	Response	Value
Eye opening	Spontaneously	4
	On verbal command	3
	On painful stimuli	2
	No response	1
Verbal responses	Oriented and talks	5
	Disoriented and talks	4
	Inappropriate words	3
	Incomprehensible sounds	2
	No response	1
Motor Responses	Obeys verbal commands	6
	Localizes pain	5
	Flexion-withdrawal	4
	Abnormal flexion (decorticate)	3
	Abnormal extension (decerebrate)	2
	No response	1

Heart sounds show normal S1 and S2 without murmurs, gallops, or rubs. Pulse is 122 beats per minute. The abdomen is obese, nontender, and nondistended, with no evident trauma. The pelvis is intact. There is an obvious fracture to the left midshaft femur. No other obvious trauma to the lower or upper extremities is found. A brief neurologic survey reveals purposeful eye movements that are equal bilaterally, and pupils that differ in size by about 1 mm (smaller on the right) but are equally reactive. The patient is rolled to evaluate the posterior trunk; no obvious wounds or injuries are found. Two large-bore IV catheters have been established, and blood has been sent to the lab. The patient's blood pressure is 90/60, respirations are 26 and slightly labored, pulse is now 130 with the cardiac monitor showing sinus tachycardia and occasional premature ventricular conductions (PVCs). His rectal temperature is 97.8°F. His O_2 saturation monitor reads 76.

T A S K S

1. What should you do now?

2. Identify the problems that need attention in order of priority. Consider the EKG and O_2 saturation readings—what do they indicate? What may affect the accuracy of the O_2 saturation reading?

3. Discuss or consider the mechanisms of those problems.

4. Are there medical or nontrauma problems you should consider?

5. What x-rays and other diagnostic studies should you consider at this point?

6. How should x-rays be taken?

7. Should drug screening be done? If so, for what drugs should the patient be screened? What is required for a drug screen at your institution? How long before the results are available?

Author's Note: One of the most important parts of evaluating a trauma patient is to know how the injury happened (mechanism of injury) so that you may consider the severity of injuries and prior conditions (e.g., inebriation) that otherwise might not be considered. Appropriate tests for this patient include a test of blood alcohol level and a drug screening. Additionally, you may want to do a quick blood sugar test if the laboratory results are delayed.

T A S K

List the steps of the secondary survey, and describe what you are looking for.

SECONDARY SURVEY

During the secondary survey, you find the following:

- Scalp laceration is still bleeding.
- Pupils are still unequal as described before.
- No facial trauma (e.g., broken nose, missing teeth) is evident.
- There is no bruising behind the ears and no blood behind the tympanic membranes (TMs).
- At the neck, the trachea is still midline, with veins flat.

- Lung sounds clear to auscultation on the right and upper left, absent on lower left.
- The abdomen is slightly obese but not distended. Bowel sounds are hypoactive. Abdomen is nontender to palpation.
- The pelvis is stable, with no blood at the urethral meatus.
- Rectal exam reveals normal sphincter tone, normally placed prostate, no masses, and no frank or occult blood.
- The left thigh is markedly edematous with tight, shiny skin and outward angulation. Peripheral pulses are weak, intact, and equal bilaterally.
- A portable, cross-table lateral x-ray of the cervical (C) spine shows no dislocation or fracture.
- A portable anteroposterior (AP) x-ray of the chest reveals a left hemopneumothorax with fractures to ribs 6 to 8.

T A S K S

1. What are the causes of each finding?

2. List the interventions for each finding (tubes placed, IVs, medications, etc.).

3. List the steps for these interventions and the contraindications for each.

4. What is the value of the C-spine films? When are they done? Why are they done? What does it mean as you progress in treatment?

The scalp bleeding should be controlled with Raney clips. A chest tube, gastric tube, and Foley catheter should be placed. The fractured femur should be stabilized.

T A S K S

1. List the possible causes of this patient's weakened pulses and decreased blood pressure.

2. What are the signs and symptoms of shock? What is the definition of shock?

3. List the different types of shock.

4. List each injury in this patient that could lead to shock.

5. What are the treatments for shock?

6. What are the results of shock to vital organs if treatment is delayed?

LABORATORY TESTS AND DIAGNOSTIC STUDIES

1. The abdominal and pelvic x-rays are normal.
2. The blood alcohol level is 0.01, and the drug test result is negative.
3. Blood sugar is 76.
4. All other study results are within normal limits. Urinalysis (UA) reveals no blood.

The patient has had 2 L of warmed crystalloid fluid with the following results: Pulse 96; Respirations 20; Temperature 98.4°F (rectal); Blood pressure 104/76.

The patient has started answering questions somewhat appropriately but is still sleepy. His blood pressure has increased and his pulse has decreased, indicating stabilization with the fluids.

T A S K S

1. What is the patient's Glasgow Coma Scale score now?

2. Should you evaluate the abdomen further for internal bleeding? If so, what tests should you consider? What test or tests give the most reliable results? (The hospital you are working at has a computed tomography (CT) scanner, but currently it is not working.)

3. How much blood does a person have to lose to cause a significant change in the complete blood count (CBC)? How long does it take for the CBC to change?

The discussion now should center on what the next appropriate action should be. This small hospital has no trauma surgeon.

T A S K S

1. Should the patient have a CT scan of the head in light of his pupillary findings, even though his Glasgow Coma score has improved?

2. Should the patient be sent to a trauma center? Is his condition stable enough for transport?

3. What are the criteria for a patient transfer in your area?

4. What are the criteria for a transfer using a helicopter?

5. At what point should you notify your supervising physician about the patient? Review your state statutes, rules, and regulations.

GENERAL DISCUSSION

The key to good emergency care is attention to detail, logical progression of evaluation, and treatment to save a life first and then to prevent morbidity. Always expect the worst. Patients suffering from trauma and other emergencies need repeated evaluation. Some very serious conditions (e.g., ruptured spleen) do not manifest themselves early in the post-injury period. If the patient does not improve with initial, standard treatment, look for the unusual, hidden or less obvious problems, pre-existing conditions, etc. Stay up to date on the BLS, ACLS, and ATLS.

Resource Notes

List all the references you used for this case.

"I Feel Tired All the Time."

J. DENNIS BLESSING, PhD, PA-C

BACKGROUND

You are working in a large, multispecialty internal medicine clinic in a large midwestern city. Many of your patients come from or are referred from outlying rural areas.

PATIENT HISTORY

Paul Toms is a 78-year-old, white, retired seaman who lives alone in a small town about 125 miles from your practice. He was in generally good health until age 73 (5 years ago). At that time, he was admitted to a small hospital in a town near his home. His admitting diagnosis was acute congestive heart failure (CHF). After stabilization of his condition, he was transferred to your hospital. An admitting resident obtained an essentially negative past medical history, except that Mr. Toms admitted to being diagnosed with hypertension at age 45. Over the next 10 years, he intermittently took assorted medications and saw various physicians when he felt like it, but by age 55 he had stopped all medications. He denied any symptomatology related to hypertension and target-organ disease. He has led a "healthy and vigorous" life. His hospital course was uneventful.

Evaluation during his hospitalization revealed the following: cardiomegaly with an ejection fraction of 50%, evidence of an old posterior myocardial infarction (MI) on electrocardiogram (EKG), early emphysematous changes on chest x-ray, benign prostatic hypertrophy (BPH), mild to moderate hypertension controlled by medication, and mild hyperlipidemia. His discharge medications were digoxin, 0.25 mg once daily; furosemide, 40 mg twice daily; potassium, 10 mg twice daily; terazosin, 2 mg at bedtime; and enalapril, 10 mg once daily.

He has come to your practice each year since that hospitalization for routine follow-up, seeing a different provider each time. His medications have been continued, and routine laboratory tests have been conducted with no abnormalities noted. He tells you that he sees a couple of "other docs" when he needs to or when he needs his medications refilled. These providers practice near his home.

His current complaints are that he feels weak, lethargic, and run down. He adds that he has no energy, is sleeping a lot, and has an irritating cough.

T A S K S

1. Develop a list of diagnoses based on the preceding history.

2. Based on the patient's current complaints, develop a list of possible complications related to aging, his illnesses, and his medications.

3. What is the current thought on treatment of CHF, with consideration to the patient's other known problems?

4. What additional history do you want? Review the components of an interval history. What are the components of the periodic examination for the patient's age group?

5. What would be the pertinent physical examination (PE) based on the history?

6. Begin to think about what diagnostic tests you may want.

ADDITIONAL HISTORY

Mr. Toms states that he has generally done well since his last visit. He faithfully keeps his annual appointments because he believes your quality of care is the best. He says that it is also a way for him to check that his other providers are doing the right things. A physician assistant (PA) in a rural health clinic in his town provides his health care; the PA works for a doctor in a nearby larger town. Mr. Toms will occasionally go to an acute care clinic in a suburb of your city. During the past year, he has also gone to the emergency department at a hospital in your city for bronchitis.

He generally sees the PA every 6 to 8 weeks, primarily for checks of his blood pressure (BP). The PA has prescribed nadolol, 40 mg once daily; hydrochlorothiazide, 25 mg once daily; and a liquid multivitamin. Mr. Toms takes diazepam, prescribed by the PA's supervising physician, to help him sleep. Mr. Toms has not told the PA about his visits to your practice because he does not want her to be angry with him for going somewhere else. He takes all his medicines as directed, except for the diazepam, which he takes whenever he wants, especially when he feels "nervous." Sometimes he takes no diazepam; other times he takes 5 or 6 pills a day.

His current complaints of feeling lethargic, run down, and tired and of sleeping a lot began about a month ago. He has no pain, muscle weakness, palpitations, problems eating, shortness of breath (unless he has to climb many stairs), gastrointestinal (GI) complaints, or melena. His review of systems (ROS) is noncontributory except for the following: nocturia three to four times each night; some difficulty starting and stopping his urinary stream with dribbling; a cough productive of clear to white sputum daily, which is worse in the morning.

He has smoked two to three packs of nonfiltered cigarettes each day since he was 15. He drinks one or two beers on the weekends and enjoys an occasional shot of whiskey or tequila.

He cannot understand why he feels "so bad" when he does everything his doctors tell him. He is very worried that he will be unable to participate in an upcoming hometown festival. He wants to be ready for it because he has a dance to attend "with a widow that I have my eye on."

T A S K S

1. Revise your list of diagnoses based on the information you now have.

2. List *all* his medications, and discuss their indications, dosages, and adverse and side effects.

3. What areas of the PE are particularly important based on the history?

PHYSICAL EXAMINATION

Vital signs: Pulse 60, regular and bounding; Respirations 16, regular; Temperature 98.6°F (oral); Blood pressure 150/92; Weight: 160 lb; Height: 5'10"

HEENT: Normocephalic, atraumatic; pupils equal, round, reactive to light and accommodation (PERRLA); arcus senilis present bilaterally; extraocular movements intact (EOMI); conjunctiva clear; sclera white; optic disc flat with bilateral venous pulsation; no exudate or hemorrhages but mild arteriovenous (AV) nicking; auditory canals patent; tympanic membranes (TMs) intact, whitish-gray, in neutral position with visible landmarks and cones of light, and mobile; cannot hear whispered voice but can hear low normal speaking voice; Weber midline; Rinne AC>BC; nose patent; mouth edentulous; pharynx with no lesions, posterior erythema, or exudates; neck supple without adenopathy; low-grade bruit in the right carotid; thyroid nonpalpable

Chest: Symmetrical expansion; hyperresonance on percussion; breath sounds coarse without rales, rhonchi, or wheezes; diaphragmatic excursion 3 cm bilaterally; heart sounds loud but with a normal S1 and S2 and no murmur, gallop, or rub; apical and peripheral pulses correlate

Abdomen: Active bowel sounds in all four quadrants; flat; nontender; 1/6 bruit over aorta; no pulsatile masses

Extremities: No clubbing or edema; toes cool to touch and a reddish-purple color that is dependent; skin from the midtibias to ankles brownish and slightly scaling; dorsalis pedis (DP) and posterior tibia (PT) pulses are 1+/4; capillary refill 4 seconds

Musculoskeletal: Full range of motion (FROM) across all joints

Neurological: Oriented to person, place, and time; responds appropriately; can perform gaits; reflexes 2+/4 at biceps, triceps, patellar, and Achilles; plantar reflex down; vibratory sense intact at wrist and ankles; stereognosis and sharp/dull intact; cranial nerves III–XII grossly intact

Mini-Mental Status Examination score: 26

Geriatric Depression Scale (short form) score: 3

T A S K S

1. Based on the history and PE, revise your list of diagnoses.

2. List the laboratory tests and diagnostic studies you want to obtain.

3. List the benefit or what you hope to discover from each test you order.

4. What do these tests cost? Will Medicare pay?

5. What are the Mini-Mental Status Examination and Geriatric Depression Scale? What do the results mean?

LABORATORY TESTS AND DIAGNOSTIC STUDIES

1. Complete blood count (CBC) result is within normal limits.
2. Electrolyte levels are as follows: sodium 140 mEq/L; potassium 2.9 mEq/L; chloride 100 mEq/L; bicarbonate 27 mEq/L.
3. Creatinine level is 2 mg/dL.
4. Blood urea nitrogen (BUN) is 30 mg/dL.
5. Glucose is 150 mg/dL.
6. Thyroid-stimulating hormone (TSH) is 8 μU/mL.
7. Urinalysis shows glucose 1+, protein 1+, and remainder within normal limits.
8. Your EKG today shows: rate is 60 with occasional premature ventricular contractions (PVC) (two seen on 30-second strip), flat T waves, U wave present, borderline ventricular hypertrophy, and Q waves in posterior leads.
9. Today's chest x-ray is presented in Figure 15–1.

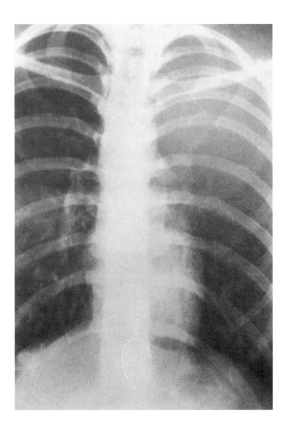

FIGURE 15–1 Chest x-ray of a 78-year-old man who complains of feeling tired.

T A S K S

1. Based on your institution's laboratory, which results are abnormal?

2. Revise your list of diagnoses. Compare your list to the one developed by the author (see Table 15–1). Remember, answers are not "right" or "wrong"—you may have thought of possibilities that the author did not consider.

3. Based on the information you have, develop a treatment plan for this patient.

4. What are the immediate problems (problems you must correct now)?

5. What are not immediate problems (problems you can solve over time)?

6. Does Mr. Toms need to be hospitalized?

7. What are his needs as an older adult, especially at home?

TABLE 15–1 LIST OF POSSIBLE DIFFERENTIAL DIAGNOSES

1. Hypokalemia
2. Diazepam abuse
3. Emphysema
4. Polypharmacy
5. Poor compliance
6. Poor coordination of care
7. Hypertension
8. Congestive heart failure
9. s/p Myocardial infarction
10. Coronary artery disease
11. Atherosclerotic vascular disease (peripheral vascular disease)
12. Hyperglycemia (Does he have diabetes?)
13. Mild renal insufficiency
14. Social situation problems
15. Tobacco abuse
16. Alcohol abuse
17. Depression (Is he depressed about living so far from the ocean?)
18. Poor or inadequate nutrition (no teeth)

GENERAL DISCUSSION

Author's Note: Remember, these problems have many approaches. The author's approach is not the only one. This case is not a test for which you will be right or wrong (unless you do something dangerous or not indicated). It is your approach and the process you follow to arrive at a reasonable conclusion that matters.

1. Take immediate action: Correct hypokalemia; should the patient b hospitalized?
2. Manage his medications (very important).
3. Ascertain cardiac status.
4. Evaluate possible diabetes mellitus (DM) and renal insufficiency.
5. What behavioral changes regarding his smoking, drinking, and diet will xyou discuss and try to promote through patient education? Will the patient make those changes at his age?
6. What would be the key points of good patient education, so he can manage his problems and make informed choices?
7. What are your plans for follow-up that include his other providers?
8. Identify who will primarily manage this patient's health care.
9. Improve communications among the involved parties—yourself, the patient, and his local providers. He should have a primary care provider who oversees and coordinates all his care. This is very important.
10. Discuss a living will, durable power of attorney, and so forth.
11. Consider home health services.

Resource Notes

List all the references you used for this case.

"I'm Having My Baby!"

J. DENNIS BLESSING, PhD, PA-C • BARBARA A. LYONS, MA, PA-C

BACKGROUND

You work in a family medicine practice that includes obstetric care.

PATIENT HISTORY

Norma Octavio, a 37-year-old Hispanic woman, presents to your office G2-P1-Ab0-LC1 at 32 weeks' gestation. She complains of uterine contractions for the past 2 hours. Mrs. Octavio has been an established patient in your clinic, and you have followed her since the diagnosis of her pregnancy at 8 weeks' gestation.

Authors' Note: Assume that the patient has complied with her evaluation regimen during the pregnancy and that the pregnancy has been normal to date.

T A S K S

1. What additional historical information should you obtain?

2. What is the general periodic evaluation schedule for pregnancy?

3. What laboratory tests are done during the course of the pregnancy and when?

4. What do "G," "P," "Ab," and "LC" mean?

5. What are the definitions of "high-risk" pregnancy?

ADDITIONAL HISTORY

Mrs. Octavio felt well until today, having no problems with this pregnancy until now. She had no problems with her previous pregnancy, which was a spontaneous vaginal delivery (SVD) at 40 weeks' gestation; she gave birth to a 7-lb, 10-oz daughter. With Mrs. Octavio's current pregnancy, she began prenatal care at 8 weeks' gestation, has followed all instructions and kept all appointments, and takes prenatal vitamins with iron. Her family history is positive for hypertension (father and brother) and type 2 diabetes (mother). Her sister was pre-eclamptic with her last pregnancy. Currently, the patient denies fever, chills, and fluid leakage or bleeding from the vagina. She says that a white vaginal discharge has slightly increased, but she has noticed no related symptoms. She has had mild nausea over the past week but has ignored it. She has had no vomiting or diarrhea. She had intercourse two nights before with no problems. Her pregnancy was advancing as expected with LMP/EDC consistent with gestational age as determined by ultrasound at 24 weeks' gestation and last fundal height measurement. She is concerned that something may be wrong with this pregnancy because of the contractions.

She complains of some occasional constipation and mild dysuria. She has noticed an increased urge to urinate but thinks that the pressure of her uterus against her bladder is causing it. (This happened with her last pregnancy as well.) She urinates every 1 to 2 hours, sometimes producing small volumes. She has not changed her oral intake. She has had some low back and lower abdominal pain for the past 2 days. The contractions feel like a tightening in her abdomen and were similar to her first labor contractions during her first pregnancy. They have come approximately every 10 minutes for 2 hours. The time between contractions may have changed slightly, but she is unsure. She has no allergies.

T A S K S

1. What is EDC, and how do you calculate it?

2. What is the significance of the patient's having had intercourse two nights ago?

3. What are the pertinent components of the physical examination (PE)?

4. What laboratory or other studies would you order?

5. What are the risks to the fetus if delivery occurs now?

PHYSICAL EXAMINATION

General: Well-developed, well-nourished woman is gravid and anxious.

Vital signs: Pulse 96; Respirations 16; Temperature 100.4°F (oral); Blood pressure 138/88; Weight 144 lb; Height 5'2"

Lungs: Clear to auscultation and percussion

Heart: Rate 96, regular; normal S1, S2 without murmur, rubs, or gallops

Abdomen: Gravid; active bowel sounds (BS); mild suprapubic tenderness without rebound or guarding; fundal height, 32 cm; active fetal movement; fetal heart rate 144 beats per minute in right lower quadrant (RLQ); contractions during examination timed by nurse at 8 minutes

Pelvic: Thin whitish discharge; cervix closed with no bulging or fluid leak

Rectal: Small hemorrhoids on inspection; no digital rectal exam done

Extremities: Lower extremities mild 1+ pitting edema, midtibia down

Neurologic: No sensory, functional, or mental deficit

LABORATORY TESTS AND DIAGNOSTIC STUDIES

1. Urine is a hazy color.
2. Specific gravity (SG) is 1.020; pH is 7.0.
3. Nitrite test result is positive; leukocyte esterase result is 3+.
4. White blood cells (WBCs) are too numerous to count.
5. Red blood cells (RBCs) are 6–8 per high-power field.
6. Bacteria many; epithelial cell = 3–5.

T A S K S

1. Is this active labor?

2. What is your list of diagnoses?

3. What is the risk of delivery now?
   A. What is the risk to the fetus?
   B. What is the risk to the woman?

4. Should the patient be admitted to the hospital or be managed as an outpatient?

5. What are the treatment options? Discuss the risks and benefits of each.

6. How should the patient be treated? Be sure to include medications, supportive care, and patient education.

7. If you choose outpatient treatment, when should follow-up occur?

8. What is the expectation for the course of this pregnancy?

9. Can this problem recur?

10. Investigate and discuss the following:
   A. Pre-eclampsia
   B. Eclampsia
   C. Gestational diabetes
   D. Abortion (spontaneous and therapeutic)
   E. Stillbirth
   F. High-risk pregnancy
   G. Birth control options
   H. Indications of fetal maturity
   I. Indications for cesarean section (C-section)
   J. Prenatal care
   K. Postnatal care
   L. Health promotion habits during pregnancy
   M. Family planning

Resource Notes

List all the references you used for this case.

"Your Son Has Been Killed."

RICHARD R. RAHR, EdD, PA-C • VIRGINIA A. RAHR, EdD, ANP

BACKGROUND

This special problem-based case examines the sudden death of a 16-year-old boy following a head-on motor vehicle collision. You, the family practice clinician, must inform the teenager's family about his death. As the clinician, you are responsible for the method, facts, and follow-up care.

Authors' Note: This case is different from other cases in the book. It is written with the hope that it will help you to begin to plan how you will deal with one of life's most difficult situations. As you work through the case, consider how you will handle working with the family, and most important, consider your own emotions and feelings. Introspection about this aspect of death and dying is very important in your development as a health-care provider.

Participants

- *Son killed:* John Robbins, 16 years old, a student at West Side High School
- *Mother:* Katherine Robbins, 44 years old, a secretary at Brown's Insurance Agency
- *Father:* Samuel Robbins, 50 years old, an engineer who owns his business
- *Girlfriend:* Michele Brown, 16 years old, an honor student at West Side High School

Information

It is a cold Friday in March. At 1:30 PM, emergency department (ED) personnel call Katherine Robbins to come to the ED because her son, John, was involved in a motor vehicle collision. You had assisted with attempts to resuscitate John, and now you must inform Mrs. Robbins of her son's death.

John had decided to go home from school for lunch as he usually did each day. Mrs. Robbins was waiting for him after he had called her from his cell phone to say he was on his way. John was a popular student with very high grades. He played on the Fighting Tigers football, basketball, and baseball teams and was considered the best athlete in the school. He was an active member of the debating team, where he met his girlfriend, Michele Brown, during their freshman year. They fell madly in love. She is an honor student, cheerleader, and basketball and softball star at West Side. John and Michele were planning to go to Capital City for a debate team match on Saturday, and both were looking forward to the trip. Both sets of parents were excited about their children's accomplishments.

John and Michele were planning to get engaged after high school and married after college. They had both sent for information and applications to Texas A&M University. They both wanted to become aeronautical engineers. John's father has his own engineering firm and had attended Texas A&M. John wanted to follow in his father's footsteps; Michele wanted to go wherever John was.

John was killed by a truck driver who had arrived in town at 8:30 that morning after a long, all-night haul. After checking his load, the truck driver went with friends at 11 AM for a few drinks. He had not slept for two nights. After leaving the bar about noon, the driver fell asleep on the interstate highway that runs through town. He crossed the highway median, colliding head-on with the car that John was driving. John was killed instantly. He sustained multiple traumatic injuries, including an open head wound and a severe crushing chest injury from the impact of the steering wheel.

John had not been wearing his seat belt, and his car did not have air bags. He was squeezed between the seat and the motor. John was almost unrecognizable. Paramedics had attempted resuscitation, but it was obvious on arrival that there was no hope. A short resuscitation effort was undertaken in the ED. After death was pronounced, the chief physician ordered x-rays to verify the extent of the injuries to the head, long bones, and pelvis for medical-legal reasons.

The truck driver was also fatally injured and died prior to arrival in the ED. There is a strong suspicion that he was intoxicated, and a postmortem examination is being conducted. The police report that both vehicles were traveling at high rates of speed, well above the posted 55 mile per hour limit.

Joan Kennon, a close friend and neighbor of the Robbins family, drives Mrs. Robbins to the ED. Samuel Robbins is out of town, attending a professional meeting in New York City.

T A S K S

1. Consider how you would tell Mrs. Robbins about her son's death. Map out a strategy for the interaction when she arrives at the ED. Be sure to address the following:
   A. What is the first thing to do before you meet with Mrs. Robbins?
   B. Where should the interaction occur?
   C. Anticipate (and list) what questions she will likely ask.
   D. If you had been the person to call her to come to the ED, how would you have done so? Should you tell Mrs. Robbins that her son is dead before she drives to the hospital?
   E. How many details should you give regarding the extent of John's injuries?
   F. How should you respond if she asks whether he suffered greatly before he died?
   G. What persons should you have in reserve to help with Mrs. Robbins's needs?

2. How will you contact her husband, who is out of town?

3. Should you assume responsibility for telling her husband?

4. Whom could you use as a resource for telling Mr. Robbins in New York City?

5. What are different ways Mr. Robbins could be told about his son's death?

You inform Mrs. Robbins of her son's death with very descriptive details of the crash. You answer all her questions. This takes about 1 hour. Next you need to deal with some very immediate issues and decisions.

T A S K S

1. Would you take Mrs. Robbins to see her son?

2. How would you inform Mrs. Robbins of the need for an autopsy on her son because of legal reasons? Are there medical reasons for obtaining an autopsy?

3. Would you ask her about organ donation from her son? If so, how?

4. Would you ask her about the funeral arrangements?

5. Would you arrange for John's girlfriend, Michele, to find out about his death? If so, how?
   A. Is that part of your responsibility?
   B. Does the fact that Michele is not a member of the immediate family influence you?

6. Should you contact John's school? Is that part of your responsibility?

7. What role do the police have in this case? What should be your interactions with them if they have questions about John and your evaluation?

8. Should you let Mrs. Robbins drive herself home? (Her friend had to leave to pick up her own son at school.)

9. Would you offer sedation to Mrs. Robbins for a few days, so she can rest during this trying time?

10. Should you prescribe antidepressants for her?

11. Would you call her minister, priest, rabbi, or the hospital chaplain to see her now?

12. What are the policies of your institution or local hospital on death notifications?
    A. What are the policies for dealing with law enforcement agencies?
    B. What are the policies for dealing with attorneys?

One of the ED nurses drives Mrs. Robbins home, where she will need follow-up care. She is devastated but is not hysterical.

T A S K S

1. What would you do for follow-up care for the Robbins family?

2. Who will notify the Robbins family of the autopsy results?

3. Will you attend John's funeral? (Assume all family members were patients in your clinical practice.)

4. Discuss your feelings about the death of loved ones. Discuss your feelings about your own death. What personal experiences have you had with death, such as the death of a parent, grandparent, close relative or friend, or even a pet?

5. Share your experiences involving a patient who had a chronic illness and subsequently died.

6. Share your personal experiences with sudden death. Explore how you feel now about the sudden death of someone who was your family member or friend. Explore and discuss how you felt at the time and how you reacted. Try to remember and analyze how others, particularly health-care providers, interacted with you. Discuss what helped and what did not help. Try to identify actions that could have been done differently.

7. Discuss guilt and grieving. Sometimes people feel guilt because of things they perceive that they should or should not have done. How do you deal with this?

8. Research, read, and develop an understanding of the stages of death and dying.

9. Read *On Death and Dying* by Elisabeth Kübler-Ross.[1]

GENERAL DISCUSSION

The important issues related to sudden death in patient care are often neglected in educational curricula for many reasons. One reason is that this topic is very painful. Sudden death is by far the most difficult emotional upheaval in life because those left behind have no time to prepare for their loss. There is no perfect or exact way to gently tell a person about the loss of a very close loved one. A plethora of issues, tasks, and topics needs to be addressed and considered when dealing with this experience.

You must consider the personal side first. Often, you also must consider the surrounding circumstances such as the need for an autopsy, organ donation, and legal requirements. You must consider allowing the family to view the person, express normal grieving and hysterical responses, and make funeral arrangements. The reason this book presents this case is to allow you to consider these aspects and to practice telling persons about the loss of a close and loved person.

When the task at hand is telling a person that someone very close to him or her (child, parent, spouse, sibling, close friend) has died suddenly, the facts surrounding the sudden death must be very clear. The person hearing about the sudden death will want to know how the person died and if he or she was in great pain before it happened. Ministers, social workers, hospice staff, and community support groups can be great resources when dealing with sudden death. All persons experiencing grief involving the sudden death of a close relative or friend need gentle support and understanding during the acute phase of the experience. When people feel that their reason for living has been taken away, they will have great difficulty recognizing how to go on and put their lives together again. Therefore, all medical personnel must understand the emotional needs to be served in humanely telling the news of sudden death and giving proper follow-up care. You must learn to be prepared for responses that range from disbelief to anger.

Research from the Harvard School of Medicine demonstrated that mothers who viewed their babies after stillbirth coped and adjusted much better than mothers who did not. Even if an autopsy was performed on the babies, the mothers were prepared for what they would see, and they fared and coped better. Incidences of depression, divorce, nightmares, anxiety, and suicides were decreased in these mothers. This research is not conclusive for all cases, but it is possible that viewing and being with the person who has died, even though he or she may be disfigured, could have a beneficial effect on the grieving process. Nevertheless, the provider must handle such a scenario gently and with support from someone like a member of the clergy or a sensitive health professional.

How much detail to give the bereaved family about the circumstances of the death or suffering that the victim experienced is an important consideration. Is hiding the facts from the family going to benefit them? No answer is definite, but if the family will learn the facts anyway, isn't it better if they come from an empathic health-care professional? If you do not know the answer to the question of suffering, be honest and tell the bereaved family that you do not know. Being painfully honest about suffering, such as in a fiery crash, is a very difficult situation. No answer on this issue is definitive, but giving honest facts with a gentle, humanistic approach would seem best. Certainly, you are in a better position to judge what to say if you know the people involved and have had a previous patient-provider relationship.

When the exact cause of sudden death is unclear, an autopsy is usually performed for medical-legal reasons. The clinician needs to discuss this autopsy requirement with the bereaved family. Your discussion of the need for an autopsy can help a family in some cases. It may be required by law, but this is seldom comforting to a family. Helping the family to understand that an autopsy may help explain some of the unknowns about a death or that the results may help in the understanding or prevention of similar events in the future can be reassuring. Your explanations and empathy in dealing with the autopsy issue will affect the way the family deals with the event. Many medical centers and hospitals have realized the need for careful handling of all sudden-death issues, including autopsies, organ donation, and funeral arrangements. Some employ individuals who are specially trained in this area, and some even have a Department of Decedent Affairs to handle all the details involving bereaved families. The health professional should use such resources but should not abdicate all responsibility for what needs to be done. In smaller hospitals and other care settings, of course, such resources may not be available.

Close follow-up of the bereaved family members after sudden death is very important. Some family members who are having a very severe grieving process may need special or more individualized attention, including pharmaceutical intervention with sedation, anti-anxiety drug, or antidepressants. This aspect of support for the grieving individual and need for medication is controversial. Some believe grieving is a natural response and no medication is warranted. Others believe that the depression, anxiety, and sleep disturbances should be dealt with by more than psychological support. The decision must be individualized, based on the person's need and your personal evaluation.

Attending the funeral of your patient who has died suddenly can be important for both you and the bereaved family. Each clinician must make this decision, but the family is likely to greatly appreciate some tangible form of support and caring. We think this is especially important when you have been the care provider for the deceased patient or other family members.

As you consider this case, think about and begin to develop an appreciation for the compassion, understanding, and caring that is needed for bereaved people. You must develop the skill to handle this type of situation and to deal with those most affected. The more you understand about death and how people (including yourself) react, the better you can help those who have suffered loss. You do not have to be nonemotional. You can grieve with the family. You will undoubtedly feel a loss when a patient dies, especially in a sudden-death situation.

Being prepared to handle sudden-death crises with skill and compassion is important. In sudden death, the empathic caring for bereaved family members is much more important than covering all the logistics items. Begin now to explore your feelings and how you will help others in the future.

REFERENCE

1.   Kübler-Ross E. *On Death and Dying.* Reprint ed. New York: Simon & Schuster; 1997.

Resource Notes

List all the references you used for this case.

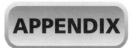

Resources for Clinical Problem Solving

BRUCE R. NIEBUHR, PhD

The print and Internet resources discussed in this appendix were selected to support effective use of the cases presented in this book and the teaching and learning aspects of the problem-based approach. This appendix does not include sources of other cases, which are widely available in both print and electronic form.

Problem-based learning (PBL) has developed in tandem with the evidence-based medicine (EBM) movement in clinical medicine. This is perhaps not surprising because faculty at McMaster University in Hamilton, Ontario, Canada, have been major figures in both areas. The practice of EBM means integrating clinical expertise with the best available external clinical evidence based on systematic research. The practice of EBM is a lifelong process of self-directed learning, completely consistent with the philosophy of PBL. Even though physician assistant (PA) students in training, particularly in the didactic component of their curricula, have limited clinical expertise, they can effectively learn how to find the best evidence from systematic reviews (such as meta-analyses) or primary studies (such as clinical trials).

PA students can learn more effectively via the PBL and EBM approaches if they have mastered the basic principles of epidemiology as it is applied to clinical practice. A minimal set of objectives for you, the reader, is as follows:

- Define and use basic epidemiological concepts:
  - Prevalence rate
  - Incidence rate

- Absolute risk
- Relative risk
- Attributable risk
- Be familiar with commonly used mortality rates:
  - Annual crude mortality rate
  - Case fatality rate
  - Infant mortality rate
- Define and use the basic concepts of diagnostic tests and screening:
  - Sensitivity
  - Specificity
  - Positive predictive value
  - Negative predictive value
  - False-positive rate
  - False-negative rate

SOME RESOURCES AND REFERENCES

Books

Friedman GD. *Primer of Epidemiology.* 4th ed. New York: McGraw-Hill; 1994.

 Many excellent epidemiology texts are available. Friedman's text is short but sufficiently comprehensive. Paperbound, it is an affordable required text for students.

Sackett DL, Straus SE, Richardson WS, Rosenberg W, Haynes RB. *Evidence-based Medicine: How to Practice and Teach EBM.* 2nd ed, with CD-ROM. Philadelphia: Churchill-Livingstone; 2000.

 This book is designed for clinicians at any stage of their education or career with a desire to practice or teach EBM. It is written for the busy practitioner: short, concise, and practical.

Barrows HS. *Practice-based Learning: Problem-based Learning Applied to Medical Education.* Springfield, IL: Southern Illinois University School of Medicine; 1994.

 This book is aimed at the medical educator, including the PA educator. It describes the PBL approach, clinical reasoning, self-directed learning, the curricular requirements of PBL, integrating other learning methods into PBL, applying PBL to clinical education, and evaluation methods.

Internet Resources

Although the Internet has revolutionized access to all sources of information, including health information, its volatility is a weakness. World Wide Web sites and links come and go. The following sites were selected in the belief that they will be fairly stable.

MEDLINE—*National Library of Medicine (NLM)*

MEDLINE is the NLM's database of references to more than 11 million articles published in 4300 biomedical journals. It is the key information resource for students, faculty, and clinicians. An important development in the history of MEDLINE is that the NLM now provides it free over the Internet to all users. Certain optional features, such as receiving copies of articles, may involve a fee.

The NLM provides alternate interfaces to MEDLINE called PubMed and Internet Grateful Med. A recent development is a consumer-oriented interface termed MEDLINE Plus. The NLM also maintains specialized databases on several topics such as HIV/AIDS (AIDSLINE), toxicology (TOXLINE), bioethics (BIOETHICSLINE), and HealthSTAR (produced cooperatively by NLM and the American Hospital Association). You can access each by navigating through the MEDLINE site: *http://www.ncbi.nlm.nih.gov/ pubmed.*

CancerLit—*National Cancer Institute*

The National Cancer Institute maintains CancerLit®, a bibliographic database specifically for cancer literature. It contains references derived from MEDLINE as well as other references to proceedings, government reports, symposia, theses, and dissertations. Available at *http://cnetdb.nci.nih.gov/ cancerlit.html.*

CINAHL—*The Cumulative Index of Nursing and Allied Health*

CINAHL®, from CINAHL Information Systems, provides bibliographic access to nursing journals and journals in the allied health science fields, including many physician assistant journals. Information in the Nursing and Allied Health database is derived from biomedical journals in MEDLINE, from nursing dissertations, and from psychological and management literature. CINAHL® is available from medical and university libraries or directly from CINAHL Information Systems at *http://www.cinahl.com.*

Evaluating Health Resources on the Web—*Moody Medical Library, the University of Texas Medical Branch*

This Web page is intended to suggest some guidelines to help both health professionals and the general public in evaluating the quality of information retrieved from Web sites. Other medical and university libraries provide similar guidelines. Available at *http://library.utmb.edu/help/evaluating.asp.*

The Problem Based Learning Initiative (PBLI)—*Southern Illinois University School of Medicine*

The PBLI is a group of teachers and researchers involved in PBL and active in faculty educational development. They provide education, consultation, and support to teachers and organizations in any discipline, profession, training program, or educational level either involved in PBL or interested in adopting PBL into their teaching or training programs. Available at *http://www.pbli.org.*

The New Mexico Partnerships for Training Project (PFT)

The University of New Mexico Health Science Center offers community-based physician assistant, certified nurse midwife, family nurse practitioner, and medical programs, using a problem-based, interdisciplinary core curriculum. The Office of Continuing Education periodically offers workshops for faculty to learn the problem-based learning approach. Available at *http://hsc.unm.edu/cme.*

Evidence-Based Internet Sites

Evidence-Based Medicine—*BMJ Publishing Group and the American College of Physicians-American Society of Internal Medicine*

Evidence-Based Medicine is an online and print journal published bimonthly. Available at *http://www.acponline.org/journals/ebm/ebmmenu.htm.*

The Cochrane Collaboration

The Cochrane Collaboration is an international group that supports preparing, maintaining, and promoting the accessibility of systematic reviews of the effects of health-care interventions. Reviews prepared using the Cochrane methods are based on the concept of meta-analysis. Look around this site at *http://hiru.mcmaster.ca/cochrane,* and browse some of the linked sites. The *Cochrane Handbook* describes how to write a review using their methods. The *Cochrane Library* is an electronic publication designed to supply high-quality evidence to inform people providing and receiving care, and those responsible for research, teaching, funding, and administration at all levels. It is published quarterly on CD-ROM and the Internet, and is distributed on a subscription basis. The abstracts of Cochrane reviews are available without charge and can be browsed or searched.

Internet Portal Sites for Medicine and Health

Portal sites are becoming very popular for patients, consumers, and health-care professionals. These sites organize health-care information and provide some editorial control over the sites. Typically, the sites offer free, public access to parts of their site and then for-fee access to other parts. Here is a nonexhaustive list of some health-care portal sites.

MD Consult

MD Consult is an online medical information service provided by a group of medical publishers. There is a fee for its use. Health-care students and professionals can "test drive" the site for free for a short time. A reduced student price is offered. Available at *http://www.mdconsult.com.*

Medscape

Medscape® describes itself as offering specialists, primary care physicians, and other health professionals an integrated multispecialty medical information and education tool. Registration is free. Available at *http://www.medscape.com.*

drkoop.com

The drkoop.com Web site is published under the imprimatur of the former U. S. Surgeon General, C. Everett Koop. The site describes itself as a consumer health-care network providing health-care content, services, and tools. Registration is free. Available at *http://www.drkoop.com.*

CONCLUSION

More resources than ever are available to help you as a student or clinician. Learn to use every resource, including expert opinion. Learn to evaluate the information you find. Erroneous information has no value and may be harmful if you accept it as accurate. You may want to develop the habit of always seeking at least two sources of information and comparing your findings. If there is conflict, seek more sources. But learn to manage the information at hand. You can be overwhelmed in your search for information. Know when enough is enough. Part of learning is questioning. The art of questioning is in finding the answer.

Index